W9-BXH-315

Classics in Psyc

A TREATISE

ON THE

NATURE, SYMPTOMS, CAUSES, AND TREATMENT

OF

INSANITY

W[illiam] C[harles] Ellis

ARNO PRESS

A New York Times Company

New York • 1976

Editorial Supervision: EVE NELSON

———•———

Reprint Edition 1976 by Arno Press Inc.

Reprinted from a copy in
  The University of Iowa Library

CLASSICS IN PSYCHIATRY
ISBN for complete set: 0-405-07410-7
See last pages of this volume for titles.

Manufactured in the United States of America

———•———

Library of Congress Cataloging in Publication Data
Ellis, William Charles, Sir, 1780-1839.
   A treatise on the nature, symptoms, causes, and treat-
ment of insanity.

   (Classics in psychiatry)
   Reprint of the 1838 ed. published by S. Holdsworth,
London.
   1. Psychiatry--Early works to 1900. 2. Psychiatry--
England. 3. London. County lunatic asylums, Hanwell.
I. Title. II. Series. [DNLM: WM E47t 1838a]
RC340.E48 1975   616.8'9   75-16700
ISBN 0-405-07427-1

A TREATISE

ON THE

NATURE, SYMPTOMS, CAUSES, AND TREATMENT

OF

INSANITY,

WITH PRACTICAL

OBSERVATIONS ON LUNATIC ASYLUMS,

AND

A DESCRIPTION OF THE
PAUPER LUNATIC ASYLUM FOR THE COUNTY OF MIDDLESEX,
AT HANWELL,

WITH A DETAILED ACCOUNT OF ITS MANAGEMENT.

BY

SIR W. C. ELLIS, M.D.

RESIDENT MEDICAL SUPERINTENDENT, AND FORMERLY OF THE ASYLUM
AT WAKEFIELD.

LONDON:
SAMUEL HOLDSWORTH, AMEN CORNER,
PATERNOSTER ROW.
1838.

LONDON:
R. CLAY, PRINTER, BREAD-STREET-HILL.

COLONEL CLITHEROW,

———

My dear Sir,

To whom could I dedicate the following attempt to afford relief to the most suffering class of my fellow-creatures, with so much propriety, as to yourself, whose whole life has been employed in promoting every scheme of benevolence, and whose personal happiness has increased in proportion to the success of your endeavours?

You have long stood forward as the benefactor, and unflinching protector of the Insane. To your influence and unwearied exertions is mainly to be attributed this spacious Building for their reception: and to your zealous and continued attention to their welfare, they are indebted for the means of procuring many of the comforts it affords. But with this, your philanthropy has not ended: you have followed them when restored to reason, and have found that they were often homeless, friendless and destitute. This was sufficient to arouse your sympathy in their behalf: you enlisted a Royal Personage in their favour ; and, under the gracious patronage of Queen Adelaide, a fund has been generously provided for their relief.

By your having kindly allowed this humble effort, for the benefit of those whose condition you have so much ameliorated, to be introduced into the world, under your auspices, you have added another to the many obligations I have already received from you, during the years you have honoured me with your personal friendship.

That your useful and valuable life may long be preserved a blessing to your fellow-creatures, is the earnest prayer of,

My dear Sir,

Your most sincere

and obliged Servant,

W. C. ELLIS.

Lunatic Asylum, Hanwell,
November 1, 1837.

PREFACE.

THE fearful extent to which Insanity prevails, the severe bodily suffering usually attending its commencement and the painful change produced by it, in the powers and moral condition of man, render it a subject of intense interest to the philanthropist and the man of science. Recent parliamentary returns show, that there are in England 12,668 Pauper Lunatics and Idiots; and the Insane alone, including the different classes of society, cannot be estimated at fewer than 10,000. From the habits and mode of education of the upper ranks, particularly of the females, the brain and nervous system are kept in a state of constant over-excitement, whilst the frame is debilitated, from the muscles being rarely called into proper and regular exercise.

Hence arises a high degree of susceptibility of disease, with little constitutional stamina, to resist the over-anxiety and other effects of the sudden changes in circumstances, peculiarly incident to the present times. Amongst the poor, different, but no less pernicious causes are followed by similar consequences. Excess, especially in the use of ardent spirits, exposure to cold, the want of the common necessaries of life, and the other results of extreme poverty all create in them a liability to Insanity. Were men, habitually, to be temperate in all things, to take no anxious thought for the morrow, and "to set their affections on things above, and not on things below," but few, comparatively, would be afflicted with this disease. Under existing circumstances, however, I am afraid that it would be enthusiasm to hope that its prevalence will be greatly diminished. The objects of the following pages are to point out the symptoms by which an attack of this disease may be foreseen, and the means by which it may be warded off; and in those cases where it has already supervened, to explain the mode of treatment most likely to restore the patient to reason and society; and where this is impossible, to show how the sufferings may be alleviated, and life rendered, if not a state of happiness at least, one of moderate enjoyment. Should the attempt, undertaken amidst anxious and laborious professional engagements, prove unsuccessful, an earnest desire to promote the welfare of a large and much enduring class of my fellow-creatures, who cannot plead their own cause, must be my apology for having made it.

Though my attention, from early life, has been particularly directed to Insanity, and a residence in the Asylums at Wakefield and Hanwell, during nearly twenty years, has placed under my immediate care and observation upwards of 2,700 cases, I feel that I have still much to learn. Even if the general view taken in the present work be correct (as I fully believe it to be), patient subsequent investigation will be required to make the picture in all its parts complete. Should I succeed in exciting an interest on the subject at all adequate to its importance, it will soon be investigated by men of more leisure, deeper research, and greater anatomical skill, than myself. If the end be but answered, and the Insane benefited, I care not whether it be by the adoption of the plan mentioned in the following pages, or by any other means. Most thankfull shall I avail myself of any additional light that can be thrown on the nature of this obscure disease, and of any mode of treatment, however opposite to my present views, by which it may be palliated or removed.

NATURE, SYMPTOMS, CAUSES, AND TREATMENT

OF

INSANITY.

CHAPTER I.

INTRODUCTION.

THE more various the forms in which a disease exhibits itself, the more difficult it is to come to a correct conclusion as to its nature. In scarlet fever, small-pox, and many other acute diseases, we find, whatever be the constitution, similar general effects, only in a more aggravated form in some than in others. In these cases we can always identify the disease; and if we cannot immediately discover its origin, we can at least find out the mode in which it shows itself. In dyspepsia, and some other disorders, the immediate effects seem to vary with the habits and idiosyncrasies of the individual attacked; and there is consequently a difficulty in determining to what morbid affection the particular symptoms are to be traced. But in no disease do we find the same complicated and varying forms as in insanity.

In some, it is attended with the highest degree of maniacal excitement, excessive muscular strength, and extraordinary vivacity of intellect; in others, the greatest depression is found, not a word is uttered, and the patient remains like an automaton for weeks together. In some, the senses are quickened, and the sight and hearing are morbidly acute; in others, they are excessively obtuse, and the whole nervous system becomes in a great measure insensible to feeling. Indeed, from our observing, that circumstances apparently similar produce results diametrically opposite in different individuals, we might be led to conclude, that, in this disease nature is at variance with herself, and that, although in all other cases she is uniform, insanity forms an exception to her rule. A further inquiry into its nature will show us that, when fully examined, these inconsistencies do not exist; and that they are to be traced to our classing under the name of insanity a set of diseases, which really act in totally different ways, and most probably affect different parts. It will be seen, that an attempt has been made in the following pages, in the first place, to investigate the nature of insanity. The results of this investigation are offered with much diffidence. It is felt, that the theory is liable to many and plausible objections, and that it is incapable of demonstration; and it is also felt that even if the view be correct, not more than the first step has been advanced in the inquiry. If it be true that insanity is really, in all cases, a disease affecting the brain and nervous system, and that it is highly probable that the parts of it which suffer vary according to the cause, and that the disease of each part is susceptible of great modification, it is obviously a work of patient anatomical research and careful previous inquiry to point out and to classify the different morbid appearances of the brain, according to the different modes in which the disease has exhibited itself. The general result is given as that which, in spite of all the difficulties, appears the most reasonable and satisfactory.

Having investigated the nature of the disease, its causes will form the next subject of inquiry. It will be seen that, in many cases, these can be ascertained with a reasonable degree of certainty. And when it is observed, that so many apparently trifling things, affecting either the body or the mind, will produce such a diseased action in the brain and nervous system as to cause insanity, somewhat of the difficulty felt on account of the various forms it assumes will be diminished. Its perusal will be attended with one cheering effect at least: it will be seen that, in many instances, the cause is capable of removal; and that, in most, proper caution and attention to the natural constitution will enable those, who are even predisposed to the disease, to avoid an attack. It is hoped, too, that when it becomes known that mere disease of the viscera, in many cases, produces it, the painful feeling of concealment, which harasses the minds of the friends, and operates most prejudicially to the patient, will vanish; and that the disease will not be suffered to be confirmed, from a false delicacy preventing the timely application of proper remedies. It will be observed that it frequently is hereditary; but there is still no reason why, even in these cases, it may not be avoided. Of course, an individual knowing that he inherits a liability to a particular disease, ought most carefully to avoid those circumstances which will have a tendency to produce it. In these cases, the constitution should be supported by proper nutritious diet; but the constant use of stimulants of any kind should, if possible, be avoided. And such a situation in life should be selected, as will place the individual in certain, though moderate, circumstances, and not expose him to any great vicissitudes either of good or adverse fortune. With these precautions, those who have an hereditary predisposition to insanity, may in general pass through life without being attacked. And the same high degree of nervous sensibility which renders this class susceptible of disease, is usually accompanied with that mental energy and activity, which make them the most accomplished and valuable members of society.

But little is known of connate idiocy, and dissection has hitherto scarcely thrown any light on the subject. In general the brain, especially the cerebrum, is very deficient in size; but in some instances the head is well proportioned, and the contents, on *post mortem* examinations, exhibit no traces of disease. It was not thought right to pass over the subject of fatuity, without adding a warning against the pernicious habit, which appears to be a very frequent cause of it.

The Chapter on Symptoms will be found to embody a somewhat minute account of those mental and corporeal changes, which usually precede an attack of insanity. If the attention of friends were but sufficiently aroused to these premonitory symptoms, the disease could, in many instances, be checked in the onset; and in others it would, in a comparatively short time, yield to simple and easy remedies. This chapter also contains a description of the most usual mental aberrations, and of the marks by which the existence of lesion of the brain is indicated. The symptoms exhibited by suicidal patients are detailed at some length ; as the care of this class is obviously one of the most painful and anxious duties devolving upon a professional man.

Great improvements have taken place in the general condition and treatment of the insane, since the horrible and disgusting disclosures brought to light by the parliamentary investigation in the year 1814. But although they are, in a great measure, protected by the present system of inspection from gross acts of cruelty, much ignorance still prevails on the method of their treatment. Nor will this be a matter of surprise, when it is considered that the subject of insanity forms but an inadequate part of medical education. In many instances, when a professional man is called in to attend a patient in a high state of mania, the disease is as new to him as it is to the friends, and he is as much terrified as any of those about him with the violence exhibited. The irritation of the patient is increased by the excitement into which all those around him are thrown; and by the excessive confinement in which he is necessarily placed, from the want of proper and convenient means of restraint. Under these circumstances, the most vigorous means are adopted; and as the pulse for a length of time appears to indicate excessive circulation, they are persevered in, until the physical powers are exhausted, and the constitution, in very many instances, irreparably injured. So many cases have fallen under my own observation, where well-meant, but injudicious treatment, the result of want of proper instruction, has rendered all attempts at subsequent cure hopeless, that some suggestions will be found to remedy this evil: it is hoped that they will not be considered out of place.

It will be seen that the medical remedies, on which much reliance is to be placed, are but few, and that they are principally of use in the early stages of the disease. The moral treatment is by far the most difficult part of the subject. In this the most essential ingredient is constant, never tiring, watchful kindness: there are but few, even amongst the insane, who, if a particle of mind be left, are not to be won by affectionate attention. The attempt must be made day by day, and for weeks together; and no discouragement must be felt, if even then the end is not accomplished. Persevere, and the reward will follow. In many cases, there will be the delight of witnessing the gradual return to reason and happiness; in all the peace and satisfaction arising from a consciousness of having done what is right to the uttermost. The various modes subsequently pointed out, in which the patients have been acted upon by moral means, are not given as an enumeration of all which may be used with advantage, but merely as specimens, and for the purpose of exciting benevolent ingenuity.

In the Chapter on Asylums, several minutiæ are gone into, which, it is feared, will be uninteresting to the professional reader. It is, however, hoped, that it will afford useful practical information to those, under whose direction similar institutions are about to be built. Indeed, many things, which appear trifling to a superficial observer, materially affect both the comfort and the cost of the patients. It is hoped, too, that, whilst the hints it contains will have a tendency to diminish the expense of executing such buildings, an enumeration of the various requisites for lunatic asylums will remove the too general impression, that, because they are to be occupied by paupers, they ought, therefore, with proper economy, to be erected at as cheap a rate as poor-houses.

In the account of the mode in which the Asylum at Hanwell is managed, the various steps will be traced, by which the system of employing the patients has gradually increased, until, at the present, 454 out of 610 are regularly at work; and many of them at trades, with which they were totally unacquainted until they were taught them in the institution. When the system was commenced by myself and my wife, on the opening of the Asylum for the West Riding of Yorkshire, at Wakefield, so great was the prejudice against it, that it was seriously proposed, that no patient should be allowed to work in the grounds outside the walls without being chained to a keeper. Another suggestion was, that a corner of the garden should be allotted for their labour, and that they should dig it over and over again all the year round. The kind feeling and good sense of the people in the neighbourhood soon overcame these prejudices; and not only did they witness with pleasure the unfortunate patients happily engaged in their works in the grounds of the institution, but they were delighted to meet them emerging from its bounds, and, by a walk in the country, and a little intercourse with their fellow-men, preparing to enter again into society. They felt too, when bowed before that God, in whose sight all men are equal, that no spectacle could be more cheering and appropriate than to witness the poor lunatic listening with them to those offers of mercy, which are peculiarly addressed to the weary and the heavy laden. Most sincerely do I hope that similar feelings will soon operate in favour of the patients at Hanwell, and that an unfounded prejudice will not long continue to confine them entirely within the pales which surround the building.

An account is also given of the measures actually adopted for the punctual and orderly arrangement of the duties necessary to the management of so large a family. It is hoped, that those who are about to undertake the conduct of similar institutions may derive from it some assistance in the formation of their plans. A copy of the written rules given to each of the domestics is added in the Appendix. These have been gradually framed as experience has pointed out the advantage of the various observances which they are intended to secure. But, notwithstanding all the rules that can be laid down, much of the comfort of the patients, and of the probability of their cure, will depend upon an unceasing watchfulness, that those, under whose care they are placed, constantly treat them with the greatest kindness and forbearance. And, indeed, unless proper persons be selected, it is impossible to prevent acts of oppression occasionally taking place. When the harassing and irksome nature of the duties of the attendants on the insane, and the importance of those duties being properly fulfilled, are considered, it is obvious, that such an amount of remuneration should be proposed as should induce persons of character and respectability to offer themselves as keepers and nurses. And, in estimating what is a fair reward for their labour, it ought to be remembered, that their lives are constantly exposed to be attacked by those whose insanity has not diminished the influence of their evil passions, but who have sense enough to know that however violent or fatal the outrage they may commit, their disease exempts them from all liability to punishment.

A conviction that the insane of the middle and higher classes do not possess half the advantages afforded by public asylums to the poor, has induced me to add a short sketch of a system, which, I hope, will secure to them every facility of cure, with but little risk of improper detention. I know that objections may be raised against the system of proprietary asylums, by which I hope that these important ends may be attained. But I think if the medical superintendent is not allowed to have any share in the concern, or to derive any pecuniary benefit from the patients remaining under his care, it will be so obviously important to his professional reputation to use every possible means for their cure, and to discharge them as soon as they can be safely restored to society, that there will be no doubt but, under this system, the rich will, at least, be put upon an equal footing with the poor. If such a refuge were but established, to which the friends of the patients could at once entrust them with confidence, the disease would be stripped of half its terrors, and the constant succession of patients to such an institution would abundantly repay the proprietors.

A few observations are added on epilepsy and the diseases of the insane. On the former very little is yet known.

An attempt has been made to draw a distinction between moral evil and insanity. A marked difference between the two really exists, although this difference is often difficult to be determined in individual cases. I greatly fear that, in every large public asylum, many will be found morally responsible before God, as rational beings, for that vicious conduct, which is by society mercifully attributed to insanity.

CHAPTER II.

THE first question which naturally suggests itself to the mind, on entering on the consideration of this subject, is, What is insanity? Is it a mental, or is it a bodily disease? or are both the mind and the body simultaneously affected? As it is obviously of great importance to have a definite notion of the nature of insanity, we shall attempt to answer these questions in the present chapter.

Our total ignorance of the nature of the mind itself, and the little knowledge of the brain and nervous system, by which it acts and is acted upon, that has hitherto been derived from the minutest anatomical research, and the most patient investigation, will easily explain why so many contradictory opinions on this subject have existed amongst mankind. In the earliest periods, the insane were supposed to be possessed by demons; and superstition assigned to the priests the task of curing them by exorcism. Hippocrates, and other ancient writers, treated insanity solely as a bodily disease, although they differed as to its immediate cause; he attributing it to a mixture of bile with the blood; others, to a too great determination of blood to the head. Amongst the moderns it has more frequently been considered purely a mental disease, and requiring only moral remedies; though, within the last few years, the doctrine of its being a bodily disease seems again to prevail. But as a mere enumeration of the contradictory opinions of the various writers would evidently not tend to increase the distinctness of our notions; and as the proposed limits of the present work will not allow us fully to state the modes by which they severally arrive at their conclusions; we will investigate for ourselves the nature of this obscure and mysterious disease. Before we proceed, it is necessary to observe, that, we shall at present confine our attention entirely to Insanity. The different manifestations of mind arising from Idiocy, Eccentricity, and Moral Evil, often confounded with it, will be taken into consideration hereafter.

We have every reason to believe, that all living beings, from the smallest insects to the largest animals, possess such a portion of mind, or instinct, as mind in animals is usually called, as is adapted to their several conditions. Some require no more than is sufficient to direct them in the choice of food, to warn them of danger, and to induce them to procreate their species. In these the corporeal machinery is exceedingly simple. They are furnished with ganglia and plexus of nerves, but are without brain. When the powers of instinct are more extended, we find, in addition to a more elaborate development of the nervous system, a cerebral organization.

Ascending in the scale of creation, we arrive at man. He possesses a bodily organization and mental faculties, of a nature similar to those observed in animals, although much more perfect in their kind. But, in addition to these, he is endowed with higher and nobler faculties. He has, and ever has had, the capability of knowing, worshipping, and loving God, and receiving the influences of the Holy Spirit. And this distinction exists wherever man is found : at the poles, or at the equator ; in the white-skinned European, the sable African, or the American savage : and it is a distinction that can never be obliterated. What then do we observe in the formation of man, uniformly distinct from that which exists in all other animals? A more elaborate cerebral organization, and a great multiplication of its parts, many of which are not found in any other animals whatever, although there is no other part of the human body which is not, more or less, developed in one species or another. Now, in each class of animals, there appears to be a certain limit to the manifestations of mental power ; and it is exceedingly probable, that, in the individuals composing each class, there exists a great difference in their capabilities. We know that in various quadrupeds, and the higher class of animals, such a difference does exist, and in man, more particularly, to a very great degree.

In judging whether, in any species of animals, the functions are healthily performed, we naturally look at the previous habits and capabilities of the species ; and we do not consider the absence of that which is not usually found to exist in such a species, as any indication of disordered function ; nor should we think the existence of a capability much superior to that which is found amongst other species, of itself to constitute any evidence of soundness, because of the difference of their natural powers and habits.   Is not the same rule applicable to different individuals of the same species, and particularly in man? We know, from experience, that an immense difference, both in physical and mental powers and habits, from some cause or other, exists among men.   Whether this would, or could not have been obviated, by previous education, is foreign to our present consideration ; although I think there is very little doubt that differences do exist, which no external circumstances could remove.   We should be unable to form any opinion of the soundness of a limb or muscle, merely from knowing its absolute power.   The arm of a powerful man, though in a state of disease, may be able to lift a much greater weight than the perfectly healthy arm of a weak and delicate one.   Before the present absolute power then can be the test, we must know the previous capabilities.   Ought it not then to be the first object of our inquiries, in estimating the sanity of an individual, carefully to investigate what have been the previous habits and powers of his mind ; what has been the state of his sentiments and passions ; and what has been his general conduct ?   And would it not be irrational to conclude that a man, possessing great mental powers, is necessarily sane, because he is capable of performing with accuracy certain mental operations? and equally irrational to conclude that an individual, of weak mental powers, is not sane, merely because he is incapable of performing similar operations?   But should we not, in either case, be justified in pronouncing the individual sane, when the manifestations of his mind, his sentiments, passions, and general conduct, continue in accordance with the exhibition of his previous powers and habits ?   These may have been such, that the individual has been incapable of performing the relative duties of life, and he may have been idiotic or imbecile : but such cases do not come within our present consideration.

We arrive then at the general conclusion, that, independently of cases of idiocy, imbecility, eccentricity, and moral evil, which will be the subject of future consideration, man is sane, when, as we have stated above, the manifestations of his mind, his sentiments, passions, and general conduct, continue either to improve or to keep in accordance with the exhibitions of his previous powers and habits.   And this too whether the mental powers are great or small ; and whatever may have been the degree of cultivation ; and however great the difference between the individual and others. The object of our introducing the analogy between the mental powers of animals and their cerebral development, will be seen as we proceed. Let us now go on with our investigation as to the nature of insanity.

The first step in ascertaining the nature of any disease, is to find out what, if any, are its invariable symptoms, distinguishing these from all others which only occur under particular circumstances. What then do we find constantly attendant upon insanity ? That which is first, and invariably noticed, is some injurious alteration, either in the intellectual manifestations, or in the conduct, or in both.

It is quite clear, that if we can show that there is an intimate connexion between the action of any part of the human body, and the intellectual manifestations and the conduct, which are the subjects of the alteration uniformly found to exist in insanity ; and can also show, that where this injurious alteration exists, there is at the same time diseased organization, or diseased action, in such parts ; we shall have done much to enable us to come to a right conclusion on the nature of insanity. Now, can we not trace such a connexion between our intellectual manifestations and the brain and nervous system ? We have seen that in animals, where little mental power exists, there is a proportionate absence of cerebral organization; and that in man, where such mental powers are found in the highest degree, the cerebral organization is the most elaborate. Again, when in man the whole brain has become torpid, either from the effects of chronic inflammation, or pressure gradually taking place from the morbid secretion of serum, slowly distending the ventricles and membranes, an alteration takes place, and he is reduced in point of intellect to the level of the lowest animals: he is capable of taking his food, but all other voluntary action is lost, in proportion as the pressure and diseased organization increase. Now, what is the case when the brain is excited to an unusual state of activity? We find a corresponding alteration, that is, an increased activity, in the mental manifestations. In the ordinary use of fermented liquors, until, from their being taken to excess, torpor is superinduced, by a *quasi* apoplexy, the operation of the mind, the sentiments, and the passions, are quickened in the same ratio in which the stimulus increases the action of the brain. In phrenitis, where this increased action of the brain amounts to acute inflammation, the violence of the mental manifestations corresponds with the activity of the disease; and when, by cold applications and proper medical treatment, the inflammatory action is removed, the mind recovers its tone; but the intellectual powers and feelings are never completely restored, if the inflammatory action has remained unsubdued, until the organization of the brain and its membranes has become permanently injured. This is found, on dissection, to be the case in all instances where the insanity has been the result of phrenitis. Now it is quite clear, that every other part of the body may be diseased or even totally destroyed, and still, if the brain continue to be healthy, the mental manifestations will remain unaffected.

May we not then, from these instances, fairly conclude that there is a necessary connexion between the mental manifestations and the state of the brain ; and that, at all events, in these extreme cases of complete torpor and excited action, the injurious alteration which results in the intellectual manifestations and the conduct, is to be traced to the state of the brain ? And as we know that the assistance of the brain is necessary to our intellectual manifestations, to our sentiments, and to our passions, may we not reasonably infer that the injurious alteration which we have previously described as the invariable attendant upon insanity, may, in like manner, in less extreme cases, be traced to the state of the brain ? This inference receives material support from the result of anatomical investigation. In old cases, diseased organization of the brain is almost invariably found ; whilst in the recent cases there is rarely diseased organization, but the vessels on the whole surface of the brain are surcharged with blood, and clearly indicate the existence of increased cerebral action.

In carefully looking over the *post mortem* reports

of those whose cerebral organization I have examined, I find that in 154 male patients, 145 had disease very strongly marked, either in the brain or the membranes. Of the nine remaining, two were idiots from birth; one died of dysentery, another of epilepsy; the other five cases had not been insane more than a few months, and died of other diseases. Of the females, sixty-seven were examined; and sixty-two found with disease in the brain or membranes: in the other five, no disease was to be discovered. Two of these were idiots from birth, and, with one exception, the others recent cases. I would have given the particulars of all these cases; but as the object is not unnecessarily to enlarge the work, but to convey as briefly as possible the reasons upon which our theory and practice are founded, I shall only transcribe a few of them. These may be taken, as nearly as possible, as a specimen of what is generally found in cases where the insanity has been of similar duration. I should not have thought even this necessary, had not my experience been so much at variance with that of Messrs. Esquirol and Pinel, whose authority on this subject has been much looked up to, especially in France.

No. 1, at the time of death, was seventy-four years of age, and had been insane seventeen years. The calvaria were found adhering, with unusual firmness, to the dura mater; the vessels of the dura mater were very turgid; brain firm, and ventricles distended with serum.

No. 2, at the time of death, was forty-eight years of age, and had been insane two years. On raising the scalp, an unusual quantity of venous blood was found at the back part ; the cerebrum was remarkably tense and firm ; there were about three ounces of fluid in the ventricles.

No. 3, at the time of death, was fifty years of age, and had been insane twelve years. The brain was very turgid, with venous blood ; a good deal of serum was under the tunica arachnoidea, and a considerable quantity in the ventricles.

No. 4, at the time of death, was forty-nine years of age, and had been insane three years and six months. The arachnoid was generally opaque and milky in its appearance, with serum underneath it, and there was an effusion of four ounces in the ventricles.

No. 5, at the time of death, was forty-two years of age, and had been insane seven years and a half. The arachnoid was opaque, and the brain very firm ; there were two ounces of serum in the ventricles ; the parietes of which were highly vascular, and considerably thickened.

No. 6, at the time of death, was forty years of age, and had been insane upwards of three years. On cutting into the scalp, a large quantity of blood poured out; the vessels of the dura mater were very turgid ; brain very firm ; arachnoid thickened and opaque, with effusion between it and the pia mater ; there was one ounce of serum in the third ventricle; the lateral ventricles were not at all distended.

No. 7, at the time of death, was thirty-two years of age, and had been insane between four and five years. The vessels of the pia mater were turgid; brain firm; ventricles distended, containing six ounces of fluid: in the left ventricle there were three hydatids.

No. 8, at the time of death, was thirty years of age, and had been insane about five months. Excepting a turgid state of the veins, every part of the head was natural.

No. 9, at the time of death, was forty-six years of age, and had been insane about three months. The pia mater was found highly vascular, arachnoid slightly opaque.

No. 10, at the time of death, was thirty-six years of age, and had been insane about seven months. The cranium and its contents were natural.

In the cases where the quantity of serum has been particularly specified, the fluid was drawn by a syringe from the ventricles, and emptied into a graduated measure.

Since the foregoing cases were copied, the theory, that increased sanguineous action takes place on the commencement of insanity, has been strikingly confirmed by a *post mortem* examination, at which I was a short time ago present. The deceased was thirty-five years of age, and he had only been

insane a few months at the time of his death. On
dividing the scalp, a considerable quantity of blood
escaped ; on removing the dura mater, the whole
surface of the brain appeared inflamed, the minutest
vessels being highly injected with red blood ; the
tunica arachnoidea was slightly opaque, in small
patches ; the substance of the brain was firm ; not
more than the natural quantity of fluid was found
in the ventricles. It will be observed, that in some
of those cases no traces of disease in the brain could
be discovered. We cannot, however, conclude from
this that no disease in the brain existed. We know
that diseased action may continue in various parts
of the body for a considerable period, and yet not be
discoverable by any anatomical investigation. The
most skilful anatomist cannot find out by dissection
any traces of tic douloureux, cramp, rheumatism, &c.
In like manner, a man may have had, for many
successive years, attacks of gout, and may ultimately die whilst suffering acutely from the disease,
and yet no trace of it having ever existed may be
discoverable on the minutest dissection, although,
in most instances, it produces, after a time, chalky
concretions and distortions of the limbs. Now, we
know quite as little of the anatomy of the brain as
of any other part of the human body ; but we do
know that a very trifling alteration in its state will
produce the most important results ; as in apoplexy, the sudden extravasation of a small quantity
of blood causes death. It is, therefore, exceed-

ingly probable, considering the minuteness and the importance of the various nerves and fibres which are found in the brain, that, in those instances where we could not trace any disease, a more accurate knowledge would have enabled us to distinguish its presence.

We have, I think, shown, that the alteration which we have described as the characteristic of insanity, is, in extreme cases, and most probably in all instances, accompanied by diseased organization, or by diseased action in the brain.   It cannot, however, be denied, that this alteration may be combined with every variety of bodily disorder, and be more frequently accompanied by some, than by others ; nay, even, as we shall have occasion to show in the next chapter, may result entirely from the brain sympathizing with other diseased parts : but this evidently does not affect the argument.

We have purposely avoided the consideration of the question, whether the mind itself, under such circumstances, participates in the disease.   There is much difficulty in our considering that which we believe to be purely immaterial to be susceptible of disease ; and as the moral remedies, which we shall hereafter have occasion to mention, are equally applicable, whether insanity be considered a merely physical disease, or a disease partly mental and partly physical, it is not a question of practical importance. I cannot, however, refrain from noticing one or two objections to the theory, that insanity is purely a disease of the brain.

It is contended by some, that insanity is not a disease of the brain, but of the mind itself; and that, in the same way as fever is but an attendant on fractures and various bodily diseases, so the unhealthy state of the brain, which accompanies insanity, is but a consequence of the diseased mind. But, if that were the case, in the same way as fever would not of itself bring on a fracture, so, in no instance, where disease in the other parts of the body has by sympathy caused disease in the brain, ought insanity to ensue. But we know, and shall have occasion to bring forward many cases, in which the insanity arose entirely from diseased action in the abdominal viscera, affecting the brain by sympathy, and in which it was removed as soon as the viscera were restored to their healthy state, and ceased to irritate the brain. In the consideration of this part of our subject, however, there is one objection which, as it is enforced by the respectable authority of the late Dr. Halloran, will demand our attention.

The substance of the doctor's argument, which occupies several pages of his work, is, that there are cases in which insanity must be considered solely a disease of the mind, because there are instances in which it has been cured instantaneously by the operation of moral causes. As an illustration of his argument, he relates a case authenticated by the late justly celebrated Dr. Gregory of Edinburgh, " of a man who, in a fit of insanity, had determined on self-destruction, and who had escaped from his house in London with the determination of precipitating himself from Westminster bridge into the Thames. When about to complete his purpose, he was suddenly assaulted by an armed footpad, who threatened him with instant death ; this not being the mode by which he had purposed to part with life, alarm for his safety instantly seized him, to the exclusion of the hallucination which had been but the moment before predominant. Being freed from his unsought danger, he, with altered sentiments, returned to his family, fully impressed with the criminality of his design, as well as relieved from his previous perplexity."

Now, had we no instances where diseases, universally allowed to be bodily, were as instantaneously brought on and cured also by the operation of moral causes as these which are said to be purely mental, the doctor's argument might be perfectly valid. That this however does occur, is so universally admitted as hardly to need any proof. To those who have been in the habit of attending many patients subject to gout, instances must occur where they will recollect an attack having been brought on by violent emotions of the mind, particularly by the depressing passions, from some unexpected calamity overtaking them: and two cases have fallen under my own immediate observation, in which a severe fit of the gout was instantaneously cured in the first instance by terror, which exactly corresponds with the case of insanity brought forward by Dr. Gregory; and in the second, by anger. I shall record them as a confirmation of my argument.

A clergyman, between fifty and sixty years of age, who had long been subject to attacks of gout, was one day sitting in his library; confined to his easy chair by a severe fit in one of his feet: one of his daughters, a little girl about five years of age, ran against a book-case, which had been left by some workmen, who had been repairing it, in an unsafe position. It was just on the point of falling upon her, when the father, forgetting his gout, sprang forward, in great terror, to save his child: he succeeded in the attempt, and was much surprised to find, that he had lost the pain in his foot, and that the gouty attack had instantly disappeared.

The second instance occurred to the same gentleman many years afterwards. He was then labouring under so severe an attack as only to be able to be wheeled in his chair from the bed to the fire-side. He ordered the servant to bring into the room a table, which was too large to be got in at the door, except when turned in a particular manner; this the servant was unable to find out or to comprehend, though repeatedly told by the gentleman, who sat an impatient spectator of his awkwardness. At last he forgot his gout, jumped up in a fit of passion, pulled the table into the room, and was instantly cured of his complaint.

At a fire in the Old Jewry, in March, 1837, a gentleman named Saunders, who had been for some time confined to his bed by the gout, is reported to have been the first person who made his escape from the house. In these instances, the disease appears to have departed altogether, in the same manner as it leaves one extremity and immediately transfers itself to another. This is often done with inconceivable rapidity.

A case has lately occurred, which shows that gout is not the only bodily disease susceptible of sudden cure from moral causes. A gentleman, who had long been subject to asthma, and was at the time suffering under it, was unexpectedly called upon to nominate a member for parliament. The sudden excitement had the immediate effect of removing the disease, which did not return until a change in the atmosphere, produced by a thunderstorm, again brought it on.

The following case is taken from the second volume of " Medical Extracts." A gentleman of great courage and honour, who had been subject to asthma, by long service as an officer in India, was attacked with a severe fit of that disorder, during their encampments, which usually lasted from ten to twelve days. Upon the third or fourth day of his illness, when he could only breathe in an erect posture, and without motion, imagining that it was not

in his power to move six yards to save his life, the
alarm guns were fired for the whole line to turn
out, because a party of the Mahrattas had broken
into the camp ; and, fearing certain death if he
remained in his tent, he sprang out with an alacrity
that amazed his attendants, mounted his horse, and
instantly drew his sword with great ease, which
before he could not move from its scabbard, though
he had tried with his utmost efforts. *How* mental
emotions instantaneously bring on acknowledged
bodily disease, and as instantaneously remove it, I
do not pretend to know ; but as it is thus proved
that the susceptibility of immediate cure from moral
causes is not confined to mental diseases, this furnishes us no test by which we can determine whether
insanity be mental or corporeal ; and therefore there
is not any force in Dr. Halloran's objection.

The same mode of reasoning evidently answers
the argument, which is urged against insanity being
a bodily disease, from its suddenly being produced
by joy, grief, or any other powerful emotion of the
mind : as we know that each of these will not only
instantaneously produce bodily disease, as sudden
terror the gout, but we have numerous cases on
record where death itself has been the immediate
result.

We will only notice one more objection, which at
the first seems plausible. It is urged that insanity
is not a disease of the brain ; because disease of the
brain, to a great extent, may exist without it. The

objection may thus be answered. It is from our ignorance of the quantum of disease which must exist, according to the particular constitution, before certain consequences are produced. We know, from *post mortem* examination, that a disease of the lungs has existed to such an extent, as would have been attended with the most painful consequences to some individuals, and yet so far from the usual signs (not stethoscopic) of consumption being exhibited, no disease of the lungs whatever was suspected. Yet no one would argue that consumption is not a disease of the lungs. By a parity of reasoning, therefore, we ought not to contend that insanity is not a disease of the brain ; because diseased brain does not always produce diseased manifestations of the mind. Having then seen, that in insanity there is always some injurious alteration, either in the intellectual manifestations, or in the conduct, or in both ; and having shown that such alteration is, in cases of insanity, accompanied with diseased action, if not with diseased organization of the brain ; we arrive at the conclusion, that insanity is a disease of the brain, causing, or at least co-existing with, an injurious alteration in the intellectual manifestations, or in the conduct, or in both.

Let us next proceed to examine to what extent this alteration must exist, before we can pronounce an individual to be insane, according to the general acceptation of the term.

Strictly speaking, every individual who exhibits

an involuntary alteration in his mental manifestations, denoting the most trifling disorder, is not at
the moment in a state of perfect sanity or health,
that is, he is insane. But as, according to the
general opinion respecting insanity, every insane
person is totally unfit to manage his affairs, and
dangerous to society; we will next endeavour to
show, that there are as many degrees of insanity, as
there are of other diseases; and that in the same
way as some bodily diseases are too trifling to interrupt the ordinary course of a man's pursuit, so
there are states of insanity which neither require
restraint, nor incapacitate a man for the various
duties of life. The *measure* of insanity, that must
exist before an individual ought to be precluded
from all the comforts of social life, virtually consigned to a civil death, and exempted from the
punishment attendant on the commission of the
most heinous crimes, will be the object of our most
serious inquiry.

But before we proceed, I would again urge the
necessity and importance of remembering, that, to
constitute insanity there must be an *alteration*. For
a man of a weak intellect, but perfectly capable of
managing his affairs, may be taken by interested
relatives to a medical man; who, from having fixed
in his mind some vague or arbitrary standard of
sanity, to which the person examined does not
come up, will, without any inquiry as to his
previous state, or upon a hasty examination, give,

uninfluenced by improper motives, but simply from
ignorance or carelessness, a certificate of his insanity.
Again, a perfectly sane man, of ordinary, or even
more than ordinary, powers of mind, may, from
some unaccountable eccentricities, which not unfrequently accompany genius, be put into confinement
solely from the medical person not having inquired
into his previous habits. Another reason will naturally suggest itself to us, no less powerful than those
we have just brought forward, in showing the
necessity of attending to this distinction; viz. that,
from neglecting it, those, who have been really
insane and dangerous, have been merely considered
eccentric, and have not been put under proper
restraint, until some melancholy catastrophe has
been the result. This we find to be the case in all
ranks of society. The history of the last few years
will unfortunately bring to our recollection too
many fatal incidents, which have arisen from individuals, of the most exalted rank, not having been
properly confined, solely because, in their insanity,
they have exhibited intellectual powers greater than
those which are usually found amongst mankind :
although if their previous habits and capacities had
been attended to, such an alteration would have
been seen as would have proved the necessity for
confinement. And every medical practitioner will
recollect cases, which have fallen under his own
observation, in the humbler walks of life, where
families have been thrown into the deepest affliction,

from a father, a mother, or a child having become the victim of unrestrained insanity.

Let us now return to the consideration of the extent of the alteration, which must exist before it becomes requisite to treat the patient as insane. It is quite evident that this alteration may exhibit itself in various modes, both as it regards the intellectual manifestations, the sentiments, and the passions. The powers of perception alone may be affected. An individual may erroneously think that he sees various forms and substances, which do not exist except in his own imagination; but as long as his reason is sufficient to correct these false impressions, and he is himself conscious that they have no real existence, he is not a fit subject for confinement. Nay more; even if his reason be not sufficient to correct these false impressions, if they be of such a nature as not to interrupt his ordinary pursuits, or to render him obnoxious to society; as, for instance, if he imagines that he sees and converses with spirits, but is not influenced by them, it would be unjust to lock him up in a madhouse: though it is almost unnecessary to say, that it is of the highest importance that, in both instances, proper steps should be immediately resorted to, before these erroneous impressions have been too much confirmed by time to be incapable of removal. For although in the first instance these effects may be harmless, yet, viewing them but as the symptoms and result of diseased action of the brain and nervous system, which may, if allowed to continue, cause organic disease; it is evidently desirable to use the most expeditious means to restore a healthy state of action in these organs. But if the diseased perceptions be of such a kind as to render him incapable of the management of his affairs, or to make his conduct injurious either to himself or to others, confinement ought immediately to be resorted to. One or two instances will make this distinction more obvious.

O. M., a shoemaker, 48 years of age, had been subject to fits of mania, about once in three or four months, for many years. During the attacks he was extremely violent, and required personal restraint. In the absence of the paroxysms he was perfectly harmless, and he now works at his trade, being trusted with the knives and tools necessary to carry it on; but he at all times imagines that he has specks floating before his eyes. His vision is not defective, and his eyes have a natural appearance, but he invariably complains of these specks annoying him. He is gratified by having his eyes examined, and will then proceed with his work as usual. Now, had this man not been subject to periodical attacks of mania, it is obvious that he ought not to be confined merely on account of his labouring under this delusion.

A. B., a joiner, 35 years of age, became insane in consequence of loss of property. He was very maniacal in the early stage of the disease: being a powerful man, he was kept under constant personal restraint for a longer time than he otherwise would have been. At the end of twelve months, he was removed from the Hospital in which he was confined, to the Asylum at Hanwell, where he had an opportunity of employing himself in his former occupation. He rapidly recovered his general health, which had been somewhat impaired by confinement; and the only delusion which remained was, his thinking voices were always speaking to him. This had been the case for a long time; and it had been judged a sufficient mark of insanity to keep him in confinement. Finding, after some months' trial, that the man was perfectly capable of pursuing his avocation, and that however much this particular delusion might still exist, it had no bad influence on his conduct, he was discharged; and he has continued to be well, and to provide for his family for several years. From his own account, as he got into his usual habits, the sensation gradually wore away, and at last totally left him. Might not the appearance of specks before the eyes have arisen from some trifling disease of the optic nerve, or in the thalami nervorum opticorum? In the latter, it is not improbable that there was some disorder in the auditory nerve, and that as this gradually recovered its tone, the sensation passed away.

In this mode of considering the subject, it is obvious, that in determining whether or not an individual be a proper subject for confinement, it is quite unimportant to find out whether his perceptions are erroneous, solely as regards one class of things, or are generally incorrect: as in the instance we have mentioned. We need not ask whether the patient supposes he sees specks on his own eyes, or on the eyes, nose, face, or body of every one else. If the illusion does not prevent him from fulfilling his relative duties in society, he ought not to be confined; if it does, he ought.

We must precisely in the same manner apply our former test, when the judgment, or the reasoning faculties, are so affected as to render the individual incapable of arriving at accurate conclusions on one or more subjects; though it might at first be supposed, that a case of this kind could not occur without restraint being necessary.

A man whose diseased brain leads him to imagine that he possesses a peculiar talent for oratory, music, poetry, or any thing else, of which he is, in reality, ignorant and incapable, certainly, as far as regards these subjects, cannot be said to be sane: but still his notions may not be such as to make it necessary to deprive him of his personal liberty. The decision in the case of Davies proves clearly, that the circumstance of a man erroneously supposing himself a great orator, was not considered by a jury sufficient to justify his continuation in confinement as a lunatic. And why? because, at the time of his examination, he was found to be capable of pursuing his accustomed avocations with his usual ability; and, though eccentric in his thoughts and habits, perfectly harmless, and not unfit for society. The only reasons, in cases of this kind, which can justify the resorting to compulsory measures, are, that the symptoms indicate the existence of a diseased action in the brain and nervous system, requiring remedies to which the patient himself will not voluntarily submit: although, in this instance, his conduct may fairly be considered to be injurious to himself, and thus, strictly speaking, he is included in our definition. This is a case unfortunately of too frequent occurrence; for the very irritation of the brain and nervous system, which makes quiet and abstraction from all business absolutely necessary for the cure, at the same time creates in the patient an increased disposition to active exertion. The necessity, nevertheless, of employing most decisive measures under these circumstances is evident, in whatever mode insanity shows itself.

There are, however, cases in which an error of judgment, even on one point alone, makes the most forcible restraint immediately necessary;—as, for instance, when a man considers that it is his duty, and that he shall benefit society by taking the life of another, by burning down a church, or when he imagines himself entitled to another's property, to which, in his sane moments, he would have known he had not the slightest claim, and forcibly proceeds to take possession.

J. F., a butcher, about thirty-five years of age, a

clever industrious man, showed symptoms of insanity by imagining himself entitled to certain
property. At first he only spoke of it to his family
and friends; but after a time, when the notion
became more fixed in his mind, he went forcibly to
take possession, and turn the owner out of his premises. No disease being suspected, he was taken
up, and sent to prison for the assault, instead of
having proper remedies immediately applied to reduce the diseased action of the brain. It is scarcely
necessary to say, that as soon as the time of his
imprisonment was over, on the first opportunity he
made an attack again. It was not however until
after some years, when the disease was too much
fixed to be removed, that he was sent to the asylum
at Wakefield. Upon all other subjects this man
was rational. He was of an irritable temper, but
very manageable by kind treatment; was fond of
gardening, and was trusted to kill the pigs, &c. used
in the establishment.

We might pursue the same train of reasoning in
regard to those cases, where the insanity affects the
sentiments or the passions, and bring forward many
instances by way of illustration:—but it will be
evident from what has been previously said, that in
these, as in the other cases of insanity, in order to
justify confinement, there must be diseased action
sufficient either to render the individual incapable
of managing his affairs, or to make his conduct
injurious either to himself or to society.

The instances, indeed, in which an individual can with safety be allowed to go at large, when his sentiments or his feelings are affected, will not be so numerous as when the disease attacks the intellectual faculties only.   For it is much more easy to fulfil the relative duties of life with diminished powers of perception or reflection, than to act correctly when under the influence of deranged and excited passions.

In our consideration of this subject, we have hitherto had in view only those cases where there has been diseased action of the brain or nervous system, causing continued alteration in the notions and actions.   Before we conclude this chapter, it will be necessary for us to observe, that there are cases when the symptoms so correspond with what we have stated as the marks of insanity, that, but for their cause, and the shortness of their duration, the individual might properly be considered insane. Intoxication is an instance of this kind :—in the acts of a drunken man we discover not only great alteration in his views, but conduct most injurious to himself and to society, and this arising entirely from the stimulus over-exciting the brain.—But though this alteration is merely temporary, ceasing when the effect of the stimulus, which he has voluntarily taken, has gone off; to exempt him from punishment for any crime which he commits under its influence, is most reasonably considered by the law unjust.

By attending to the following distinction we shall, I think, be relieved from all difficulty on this part of our subject. If the paroxysms, however violent, result from causes within the immediate control of the individual, he ought to be amenable to the laws for his actions: if, on the contrary, they have their origin from sources entirely, or remotely, out of his reach, justice as well as humanity would attribute the act to madness, and forbid his punishment.

Having then, in the present chapter, endeavoured to show what insanity is, we shall next proceed to investigate its causes, and the modes of their operation.

CHAPTER III.

IF our theory be correct, that Insanity, in all its various forms and modifications, is in reality a disease of the brain and nervous system, the immediate causes of it may evidently be reduced into two classes:—the first class consisting of those which act primarily on the brain and nervous system; the second, of those which cause disease in them merely by sympathy.

But before we proceed with this part of our subject, it will be necessary to make some observations on the hereditary predisposition to insanity, which exists in different individuals.

That there are certain constitutions in which there is an evident predisposition to particular diseases, is too well known to admit of the slightest doubt. The natural conformation points out some persons as particularly susceptible of apoplexy and phthisis; others, again, from birth are liable to bilious diseases: analogy, therefore, independent of experience, would lead us to infer, that it is most probable that the same tendency to morbid action which exists in other parts of the body should also be found in the brain. Again; as we find that children resemble their parents in conformation of the body, in feature and complexion, and even in the colour of the eyes and the hair, it is but reasonable to conclude that there should be a like resemblance in the structure of the brain and nervous system; and that as other diseases, for instance gout, scrofula, phthisis, &c., are propagated for generations, so also should diseases of the brain. There cannot indeed be any doubt that insanity is an hereditary disease.

Out of 1380 patients, there have been 214 whose parents or relatives we have ascertained to have been previously insane. In 125 of these cases no other cause could be assigned for the disease coming on than that of its being hereditary. In sixty-five there were various moral causes, in conjunction with this hereditary tendency; and in twenty-four there had been blows on the head preceding the attack. If we had more complete information, I have no doubt but that the insanity would be found to have been hereditary in a much greater number.

It does not however follow, that the offspring of parents who have been insane should themselves necessarily become so; particularly if the insanity has existed only on one side. For instance, if it has taken place on the paternal side, the child may have inherited the constitution of its mother, or *vice*

versá.   Again; the brain of the parent who has
been insane may not have been more than ordi-
narily susceptible of disease, and yet, from either
physical or moral causes, of a very exciting nature,
insanity may have been brought on.   Now though
the same structure and constitution be inherited by
the child, still, if not exposed to similar exciting
causes, it may escape disease.   But even if the
brain of the parent who has been insane has had a
very high degree of morbid susceptibility, which has
descended to the child, yet, by carefully avoiding
every exciting cause, it may pass through life without suffering from this direful calamity.   It is very
possible that, had not the sixty-five patients in
whom the disease is said to have been brought on
by moral causes, and the twenty-four, where it was
preceded by blows on the head, been exposed to
circumstances tending to produce the disease, they
might have escaped; but the hereditary predisposition existing, insanity was the result.

On making inquiries of the friends and relatives,
we find, that there are a great many patients, in
whom no hereditary tendency could be traced, and
who have become insane entirely from moral causes.
Indeed, we are all probably more indebted for our
sanity to circumstances and to education than we
should at first be willing to acknowledge.   When in
early life the inclinations have never been thwarted,
and the passions have been allowed to remain
unsubdued, the disappointments and reverses of

fortune, which almost invariably attend every human being in his passage through this world, frequently cause such over anxiety in the mind, before unaccustomed to restraint, that it is no longer capable of abstracting itself from the consideration of the painful events; and its organ, the brain, from over exertion, becomes diseased as the consequence. When we find, then, that distressing circumstances, combined with the want of proper education, are very frequently sufficient to produce insanity in those who have no hereditary predisposition to it, how manifestly important is it for those who have the care of children, whose parents or ancestors have been deranged, to teach them from their earliest infancy, habits of self-government; and afterwards to place them in situations of life where they may have the prospect of moderate and certain success, rather than the doubtful hope of aggrandizement, with the possibility of failure!

There is at the present period a laudable anxiety to instruct children at a very early age. As far as this tends to their moral education, it is most advantageous: but I am afraid that the systems which exist in some infant-schools, will tend rather to weaken than to strengthen the brain, by too early calling forth the powers of the mind. In fact, the soft structure of the brain in infancy seems to indicate the impropriety of exercising it too much in its immature state: and how rarely do we meet with instances of those who have exhibited very precocious talents, fulfilling the anticipations of their friends in after life! But I am afraid that the intellectual powers not being eventually so strong as they otherwise would have been, is not the only mischief. The constant undue excitement of the brain, before the constitution has attained sufficient strength, will make the rising generation peculiarly liable to disease of that organ, and of the nervous system in general.

There are some cases in which the hereditary predisposition to insanity seems to be so strong, that no mode of education whatever will apparently prevent its taking place, even in circumstances the most favourable. In many cases, upon questioning the overseers and the friends of the patients, who have been intimately acquainted with them for years, as to what brought on the attack, their answer has been, " Their relations have been so before them, and we know no other reason." And upon the most careful investigation, we have not been able to discover any other cause, either physical or moral. But it is possible, that if we knew every circumstance connected with the case, some bodily complaint, too slight to have attracted the notice of any but a medical man, would have been found to have existed. Where the disease has assumed any particular form, this is also very frequently inherited, especially in cases of suicide.

Sarah T., aged forty-two, the widow of a labour-ing man, had been insane eighteen months previous to her admission. She was reported to have a strong tendency to suicide. Her mother and two of her sisters hung themselves : she had made several attempts on her own life. In a short time she improved in bodily health, and she appeared not to be so much depressed : she continued sometimes better, and sometimes very desponding, for eight months. She was watched with the greatest care, and not permitted to be alone ; but notwithstanding every effort, she unfortunately contrived to secrete herself in a bedroom, and hung herself to the iron window-frame, and was not discovered until life was extinct.

I cannot omit to mention in this place, that relatives by blood, intermarrying with each other, have a progeny prone to insanity. Why it is so, I do not presume to give an opinion ; but of the fact I have no doubt, not only from what has come within my own knowledge, but from its having been particularly noticed by Dr. Spurzheim, and others, who have paid great attention to the subject: it cannot be too generally known and guarded against.

We will now enumerate those causes which fall under our first division.

One of the most obvious of these is a blow on the head ; it injures the brain, in the first instance, either by compression or concussion. When the skull is fractured, so that the bone presses upon the brain, stupefaction is generally the immediate result ; this continues until the pressure is removed.

Very frequently, when no fracture has taken place, and stupefaction is the consequence of concussion only, the patient has recovered from it, but yet has subsequently died or become insane, in consequence of inflammation or irritation of the brain or its membranes, occasioned by the blow. It does not fall within the design of the present work to take into consideration those cases, where death has ensued from injuries of the head; but a history of one or two instances where insanity has been the consequence, will tend to illustrate this part of our subject.

Benj. K., a clever, sprightly lad, was employed as a farmer's servant, until he was 18 or 20 years of age. At this time, he received a blow on the head from a kick of a horse, which fractured the right parietal bone. The particulars attending the accident are not known; but it appears that, after the trepan had been applied, he recovered from the stupefying effects of the blow; but he ever afterwards exhibited a deficiency of intellect, and became subject to paroxysms of mania, particularly after taking an extra quantity of beer. Previously to being placed under my care, he had been for many years in the workhouse; and, to prevent his running away and begging liquor, he had been chained to a log of wood, which weighed upwards of forty pounds—the iron ring to which this log was fastened being changed from one leg to the other, when the skin was worn off by its friction.

He was a most miserable spectacle when admitted : on the removal of the chain his legs quickly healed, and with the good diet of the house, his general health was soon restored ; but no improvement ever took place in his intellectual faculties. He was occasionally subject to pain in the head, especially on getting rather fuller diet than usual. He afterwards became very stupid and somewhat incoherent; he was, however, soon relieved by the application of leeches, and a little purgative medicine. He continued in this state for four years, when he had a paralytic attack : he afterwards became fatuous, and died in about fourteen months, after having all the medical applications usual in such cases.

George T., aged 55, was admitted, after having been insane two years; but it seems he has never been perfectly well since he got a blow upon the head, by a piece of timber falling upon it ; how long before is not stated. He has been a very temperate man : attempted to cut his throat prior to admission : was in a very feeble and emaciated state when admitted, and died in three weeks.

Inspection. — Arachnoid membrane remarkably thickened, and opaque nearly throughout : here and there depressions, the size of a horse-bean, in the cortical substance of the cerebrum, where the opacity was interrupted. Much serum was found under this membrane, making, together with what was in the ventricles, about eight ounces. Plexus choroides very pale, with large and numerous vesicles : thorax natural : large intestines, full of fœces to a great extent.

It not unfrequently happens that, after the patient recovers from insanity produced by a blow on the head, the brain and nerves are left in such a state of irritability, that a very trifling exciting cause is sufficient to bring on a recurrence of the disease.

Matthew L., aged forty-five. In consequence of a disappointment in love, he enlisted as a soldier when seventeen: went first to the Cape of Good Hope, where he was five years, and was afterwards ten years in India. In storming a fort, he received a blow on the head, and fell from the wall : he was found after three days, and taken to the hospital, where he remained for some time in a state of blindness and stupefaction, and then became maniacal. After being fourteen months in that state, he was discharged, and sent home to England : during the voyage, he gradually recovered both his sight and mental powers; and, on his arrival at home in 1821, nothing but weakness remained of his former complaints. Ever since, he has been liable to short paroxysms of violent passion ; and on drinking a small quantity of beer or spirits, such as before the accident he could take with impunity, he becomes restless, has sleepless nights, and, if he continues drinking for a few days, becomes insane. His temper has always been extremely firm, or rather obstinate : on his father offering to buy him a commission in the army, after he found he had enlisted, he refused it, unless he might marry the young woman to whom he was attached. He had had several attacks of insanity previously to his being placed under my care; and he soon recovered. He has always been remarkably fond of travelling, and even now does not like to live long in one place.

As we find insanity to be the result of compression from a blow on the head, may we not trace to a similar cause some cases which are attended with nearly equal stupefaction, and which cease as instantaneously as those do which have arisen from pressure of part of the skull upon the brain, on its removal? As, in apoplexy, a very small quantity of blood *suddenly* effused, is sufficient to produce death, may not some part of the brain be internally pressed upon in these cases, by the *sudden* accumulation of a very little excess of fluid, yet still sufficient to cause the stupefaction? Is it unreasonable to suppose, that this pressure may be taken off by some internal operation, as instantaneously as that of the bone by the trepan ?

The following case will illustrate what is here meant:—T. J., a sailor, thirty years of age, was, when placed under my care, reported to have been insane only ten days; but he was said to have had a slight attack a few weeks previously, for which no cause could be assigned. His temper was naturally sullen, his habits sober : he was very taciturn, and refused his food. The pulse was natural, tongue white and tumid, and bowels costive. He took some brisk purgatives, after which his appetite improved; but he continued restless, taciturn, and obstinate : the extremities were cold, with a pulse small and frequent. Continuing in this state, leeches were applied to the temples, and the purgatives repeated : he seemed a little relieved by these remedies, but continued silent, heavy, and stupid : the eyes were not red, and the pupils but little sensible to light, and there was not any flushing in the face. Purgatives were repeated, blisters applied to the back of the neck, and sinapisms to the feet. He continued much in the same state, and perfectly mute for about a month, when he had a very severe attack of dysentery. He recovered in about a fortnight, a good deal weakened by the disease, for which the usual remedies were applied; but without the slightest change in his mental affection. During the two following months, the warm bath was ordered; and the latter half of the time, a perpetual blister was applied at the back of the neck, without producing any improvement. He was then seized with convulsions. The vessels of the tunica conjunctiva being much loaded with blood, leeches were applied to the temples, and his bowels kept open, and his usual bodily health soon returned; but his mental disorder remained unaltered, and no impression could be made upon him by any moral means. His wife and relatives came to see him, and brought with them his child; but he took no notice whatever of any one of them, and remained perfectly mute. He continued in this state for three months, until one morning when the keeper, on going into his room, was astonished to hear him inquire where he was. The patient told him, that when he awoke in the morning he found all his senses and powers of mind restored to him. He had no recollection of any event that had occurred for seven months. He continued perfectly well for some weeks, when he was discharged. During the time he was convalescent, all his old habits were resumed; he enjoyed his pipe and tobacco, and the gait so peculiar to sailors returned, and he paced the galleries exactly as he would have done the deck of his ship.

Coup de soleil is another instance of primary injury of the brain causing insanity. W. S., age thirty-five, married, and has six children; has been employed in a warehouse, and has occasionally travelled for the house. During his journey in a very hot day, he felt himself extremely oppressed with the heat, and was seized with a violent pain in the head. His father thinks he has never been perfectly well since; for though no aberration of intellect took place until about seven weeks afterwards, yet his friends perceived a little unsteadiness in his gait, and a trifling stammering in his speech. The first symptoms of derangement which were observed were involuntary fits of laughter, great and unusual rapidity of expression, and general good-tempered excitability. Temper naturally mild, habits very temperate, bowels open; he is reported to have been cupped, blistered, purged, &c., but at what period after the attack came on does not appear. He took nitre, squills, and digitalis for about ten days; he afterwards continued the diuretics, with inf. gentian for about six weeks, occasionally taking jalap and calomel to keep his bowels open. He improved very much in his general health under this plan of treatment, but very little alteration took place in his mental manifestations. He imagined that he possessed the power of instantly transporting himself from one country to another. After remaining about six months in this state he was removed home by the desire of his friends; and I afterwards learnt that he gradually became fatuous, and died in about twelve months afterwards.

G. B., age thirty-seven, single; is reported to have been insane ten weeks. He says, that in one of the hot days in August, being too late for a coach by which he intended to go, he ran a considerable distance without his hat, and was immediately seized with a violent pain in the head, and had never been quite well afterwards. Bowels regular, temper mild, habits sober, pulse ninety-two, tongue furred; imagines that he labours under syphilis, but has no symptom of that disease—is much depressed. His bowels were kept open by small doses of rhubarb, he used the warm bath three times a week, and took tonic medicines. He gradually recovered, and was discharged, cured, in three months; he continued perfectly well when the last accounts were received of him.

Amongst the primary causes of insanity we must not forget to mention old age. It seldom happens that the decay of the body is so general and uniform that some one part of it does not show symptoms of disease, while the other parts remain unaffected. In many cases the limbs give way, and lameness is the first symptom of decreasing vigour; in others, weak vision, loss of hearing, or disordered functions of the stomach or liver, announce a fast approaching dissolution. Now the brain in the same way becomes weakened and worn out; we find in the loss of memory, defective judgment, diminished reasoning powers and altered views, symptoms of its disease. The most amiable of mankind, under this afflictive dispensation, so lose the power of restraining their feelings as to render themselves unfit for the society of their relatives and friends, and to make restraint and confinement absolutely necessary. It is, however, consoling to reflect, that these painful changes are not the result of any alteration in the moral character, but solely of a disease of the brain. In all cases where we have examined the brains of those who had previously had senile insanity, considerable disease has been found.

Wm. D., aged seventy-five, has been insane two years; it appears from the overseer, that he has for some time been in an imbecile state; but, being harmless, very little notice was taken of him. He has lately been restless in the night, has wandered about for days together, and destroys his clothes. Temper sullen, habits sober. He was attacked with pulmonary disease, and died in about three weeks after admission.

On examination, the dura mater was found adhering to the cranium. Arachnoid opaque to a great extent, with here and there white patches of organized lymph, and a good deal of serum under it. Pia mater very much thickened, its arteries minutely injected, and its veins enormously distended; the membrane being so tough and firm as to allow of its being pulled out entire from the whole of the cerebrum. The brain itself very flaccid, shrunk, and exsanguineous; lateral ventricles contained about four ounces of serum; the plexus choroides had hydatids attached to both sides; septum lucidum open, cerebellum also flaccid. Some flakes of coagulated lymph were found on the surface of the right lung, and adhesion had taken place in several parts of the left lung; contents of the abdomen nearly natural.

Joshua L., aged eighty-eight, had been labouring under senile insanity between three and four years before his death. He was totally blind in the left eye, and the vision of the other was nearly gone.

On dissection the dura mater was found firmly adhering to the cranium, the latter very thick; brain soft, six ounces of serum in the ventricles; optic nerves very flat and collapsed, with great vascularity in the brain just behind them; basillary and other arteries much ossified, as well as the aorta and the iliacs. Left lobe of the lungs contained a good deal of pus.

T. B., aged seventy-eight; had been labouring under senile insanity for four years before his death. Arachnoid very opaque, firm, and nearly as thick as the dura mater; between one and two ounces of serum between the membranes, and three ounces in the ventricles. Substance of the brain soft.

Joseph I., aged seventy-five, had been insane some years before his death, the faculties having gradually declined. Arachnoid generally opaque, with serum underneath; pia mater much thickened and consolidated. About two ounces of serum were found in the ventricles.

C. H., aged seventy; reported to have been insane only six weeks; but his appearance and manner indicated senile insanity of much longer standing. There was a general diminution of the powers of the mind, with considerable feebleness of body, which daily increased. He died of chronic diarrhœa, about six months after admission.

Post-mortem Examination.—Head—cranium thin. Arachnoid opaque, and much thickened in some parts; eight ounces of serum were found in the

ventricles : olfactory nerves softened ; brain generally soft, and full of bloody points. Thorax—
four ounces of serum in the left side ; great adhe-
sions and venous congestion in the lungs, some parts
of them hepatized. Abdomen—spleen and liver
small and pale ; pancreas tubercular.

Apoplexy and Epilepsy will be the subject of
future consideration, although I am aware that they
are, by many writers, classed amongst the causes of
insanity. But as both are always attended by a
morbid state of the brain or its vessels, I think
them rather the consequence of the same diseased
action in the encephalon, (which, in some constitutions, would have produced insanity,) than the direct
causes of it. In fact, as we know that there exists
in certain individuals a liability to be attacked by
some diseases, and a great indisposition to be
affected by others, we ought not to be astonished
at the different results which take place from
similar causes acting upon the brains of different
persons.

By far the most general primary cause of diseased
action of the brain, and therefore of insanity, is
over-exertion. When the brain has been for too
long a time intensely employed upon any subject,
it is thrown into such a state of excitement that its
operations are no longer under the control of the
will : the incipient stage of insanity then com-
mences, a superabundant flow of blood is propelled

to the head, irritation and want of sleep are the
immediate consequences, and, if proper treatment
be not applied, inflammation is the ultimate result.
This diseased action, if unchecked, produces diseased organization, or that chronic state of insanity
which is attended by congestion of the vessels,
the opacity of the membranes, and serous effusion
under them and in the ventricles, so generally
found in the heads of those who have been insane
for any length of time.

To this over-exertion we must attribute an immense number of the cases arising from moral
causes; for, as the brain is the organ of the mind,
not only will an undue exertion of the sentiments
and the passions cause this irritation, but too continued thought on subjects difficult to be comprehended, or even on those which are within the grasp
of our understanding, when they interest us too
deeply, is quite sufficient to produce such over-
excitement.

Among the class of patients admitted into pauper lunatic asylums, intense study is not a usual
cause of disease.   We select the following cases:—

G. C., a very respectable young man, twenty-six
years of age, was entirely dependent upon his brother, a clergyman, who had himself but a small
income and a large family.   He was reading for
orders; and his anxiety to pass a good examination
before the bishop, induced him to apply with such
intensity as to bring on derangement.   He had

been twelve months confined in a private asylum previously to his coming under my care : he is said to have been much depressed in mind ; he appeared in a weak, feeble state. He was put on a nutritious diet, and had half a pint of porter daily ; he took inf. gentian, and small doses of rhubarb occasionally, to keep his bowels open. An improvement was very soon evident both in the powers of his mind and body. This continued for about a month, after which no improvement took place mentally for five months, when he gradually began to recover his mental powers, and was discharged, cured, after having been nine months in the asylum. He was enabled soon after to pursue his studies, and obtained ordination. When I last heard of him he was performing his duties as a Christian minister, much to the satisfaction of his parishioners.

The following case is a remarkable instance of a multiplicity of objects, not of themselves individually calculated to excite the mind, overworking the brain from their too rapid succession, and producing insanity.

M. P., age twenty-one, a single woman ; had been insane about three months. The attack came on, in a slight degree, when she was in London, where she was on a visit. The novelty and great variety of the objects presented to her view brought on confusion of ideas, which she was unable to overcome. On her return to the country this confusion continued, and she became insane. She has been very much depressed ever since the disease came on, and attempted to hang herself.   She recovered perfectly in four months.

Another female from the country, about twenty-five years of age, was in London for a short time, and was affected precisely in the same way; excepting that, instead of its producing the distressing feelings with which the former patient was afflicted, she was very cheerful, was making speeches, and acting as if she was constantly surrounded by company; and talked of nothing but the parks, theatres, squares, streets, &c. &c.   The disease coming on gradually, but little notice was taken of the alteration in her manner and conduct : no remedies were applied for a long time, and the disease was found to be incurable.

As the asylums at Wakefield and Hanwell are established solely for the reception of the poor, it will not be a matter of surprise that a greater number of its inmates, both male and female, are sent thither through distressed circumstances, than from any other moral cause.   These cases generally occur amongst married persons.   Parents, in addition to their own personal sufferings from want of the common necessaries of life, are continually enduring the most painful anxiety, from seeing their children, who look up to them for support, undergoing the same privations, without their being enabled to afford them any relief.   It is a lamentable fact, that the most frequent instances of insanity, from this cause, are amongst the honest and industrious. A poor man who has been in the habit of maintaining his family in respectability, has been, from depression in trade or some untoward circumstances, thrown out of employment, or not able with his utmost exertions to earn what has been sufficient for the bare sustenance of his wife and children. He has been unwilling to apply to the parish for assistance; or, when driven there by absolute necessity, has received such a scanty pittance from a harsh and unfeeling overseer, as barely to enable him to drag on a miserable existence, with a body emaciated from want. The brain participating in this general weakness, is no longer able to endure the high state of action into which it is thrown by anxiety, without having its functions injured.

J. P. had been a surveyor, and had a wife and large family. He was in tolerably good circumstances, until he became bondsman for a person who failed, and he was called upon to pay the money. This involved him in difficulties which he could not overcome: he gradually became so reduced, as to be at last without the common necessaries of life. The daily scene of misery created an anxiety which in a short time rendered him insane. He was in a very feeble state when admitted into the asylum, apparently from insufficiency of nourishment. Indeed, he informed me, after his recovery, that frequently not having adequate food for his family, he left his house at dinner-time, to save them the pain of seeing him fast, while they shared in a scanty meal. After a few months, proper diet, with active employment, restored him. His mind was relieved by the promise of business on his discharge. He returned home, obtained employment, and continued well.

M. A. formerly moved in a very respectable circle. During many years, by her professional exertions in music and drawing, she contributed to the support of her aged parents, and obtained a sufficiency to purchase a house, besides some trifling amount of funded property. Age coming on, she was unable to follow her employments; and, notwithstanding the most rigid economy, her little capital was soon expended. She was obliged, too, to part with her house; and the purchaser, by taking advantage of her necessity, obtained it for one-third of its value. The grief and anxiety from these accumulated misfortunes, operated so powerfully upon her active and sensitive mind, that she became insane.

M. R. formerly resided in London, and traded in ready-made baby-linen. By industry and economy she maintained herself comfortably, and, in consequence of an increased business, re-fronted the shop at her own expense. Soon after this, she received notice to quit; though the landlord had promised, when she made the alteration, to grant a lease for seven years. As he neither listened to remonstrance nor allowed any compensation, she was obliged to leave the premises, and give up business. Having no other means of subsistence, the prospect of poverty harassed her mind, her anxiety brought on excessive watchfulness, and insanity followed. She came into the asylum a short time after the attack commenced. She was in a very maniacal state ; but this having been overcome, her attention was soon attracted to some work in progress in the bazaar established in the asylum, of a similar kind to that in which she had previously been occupied. She voluntarily offered to cut out some children's caps and other baby-linen ; from this time she began to recover rapidly, and was shortly afterwards discharged cured.

J. C., about fifty years of age, once occupied a small farm, and had the management of another around the mansion of his landlord. He was highly respectable, and much esteemed by his master. During the depressed state of the agricultural and commercial interests, after the great panic in 1825, he began to lose money, and the utmost diligence and labour could not prevent his rent being in arrear. He was an affectionate father, and the prospect of a large family being reduced to poverty haunted him ; he became sleepless, restless, melan-choly, and unable to pursue his occupations, though convinced that great exertion was requisite to avert impending ruin. His family were unwilling to send him from home, and his landlord behaved kindly. As nothing could allay his irritable feelings, he was, after a long unavailing struggle, sent to the Wakefield asylum.   His head was hot, his extre- mities cold ; the stomach and bowels were disor- dered, and he had sleepless nights.   Application of cold to the head, and warmth to the extremities, with proper remedies to restore a healthy action of the chylopoietic viscera, together with his being absent from his family and all those scenes which recalled his former painful feelings, soon restored him, and he returned to his occupation.

This state of poverty, too, is not only a source from which the disease first originates, but it very frequently is the cause of relapses.   Removal from the scenes of misery which have been so painfully felt, and occupying the mind with other objects, aided by the influence of good diet, have often pro- duced very salutary effects in a short time, and ultimately restored the patients to sanity.   A return to the poverty which they had left, has, however, in many instances brought on fresh attacks almost immediately.   This is a fact that cannot be too forcibly impressed on the minds of those whose duty it is to watch over the poor.   A few pounds judiciously applied in such circumstances would often not only rescue a fellow-creature from the sufferings attendant on this disease, but, in addi- tion, save the parish the expense of maintaining the man himself, probably for life, and his family until they can provide for themselves.

Within the last few years, by the munificent

bequest of a thousand pounds from the late John Harrison, Esq., of London, to the Asylum at Wakefield, the visiting magistrates of that institution have been enabled to bestow a donation of a few pounds on patients who have been discharged cured, when their circumstances have required such assistance. The cheering influence upon the mind from the possession of such a little independence, upon which they could rely without applying again to the overseers for assistance, until they could obtain employment, has, I have no hesitation in saying, in many instances, preserved them from the immediate recurrence of the disease.

The following is a very striking case of the good effects arising from timely assistance being afforded when intense anxiety, arising from poverty, is the cause of insanity :—

G. W., aged fifty-three, a weaver, of very sober, industrious habits, but with a large family, fell into very distressed circumstances from his wages being low, and having much sickness amongst his children. These combined brought on a fit of insanity. He was admitted into the Asylum at Wakefield, and after remaining eight months, perfectly recovered. During his confinement, his eldest daughter, with most exemplary kindness and good feeling, had contrived, by great labour and the strictest economy, to support both herself and the younger children, without any assistance from the parish. But a year's rent of five pounds becoming due, they were totally unable to provide for it. The landlord threatened to distrain; and their loom, the only source of their maintenance, was about to be taken from them. The poor girl came over to relate the painful circumstance to her father, who was then convalescent; but such was the shock produced by this intelligence, that in all probability he would have relapsed, had not the money for the rent been provided. This was done, and he went home with a thankful and joyful heart.

I cannot forbear making an extract from a report of my intelligent successor at Wakefield, Dr. Corsellis. It will shew, in a very forcible manner, the great advantage derived from the fund.

" A poor woman, the mother of a large family, was admitted from the township of Leeds, labouring under the most distressing melancholy, having several times attempted self-destruction. It was ascertained that debts to the amount of twenty pounds, a sum she had no prospect of ever being able to pay, were the originating cause of her disorder. On investigation of the circumstances, the parish authorities of Leeds, with that humanity so peculiar to them, unhesitatingly agreed to allow the same sum towards liquidating the debt, as that awarded from Harrison's fund. The creditors readily accepted ten shillings in the pound, and ten pounds discharged the whole debt. The relief of mind was soon apparent in the cheerfulness of this honest creature; she rapidly recovered, and in a few months after was discharged perfectly cured."

Too intense thought upon religious subjects is the moral cause, which, next to distressed circumstances and grief, has produced, as far as we have been able to ascertain, the greatest number of cases in the institution at Wakefield.   Very few of the patients in the asylums on the Continent are said to have become insane from this cause.   This great disproportion might at first be matter of surprise; but when we see that religious discussion is in some countries forbidden, from political reasons, and that in others it never takes place, from the general prevalence of infidelity amongst the higher orders, and ignorance and blind superstitious obedience to the dictum of the priests amongst the lower classes, the mystery is easily solved.   As there are more sectarians of all kinds in England than in any other part of the world, except America, religion is more immediately brought home to the poor as a subject of thought and examination.   Wherever a variety of opinion exists, and freedom of discussion is allowed, the attention is naturally roused, and the feelings become excited.   And when the immortality of the soul, and the awful realities of eternity, are first impressed upon the mind of an individual, who has never before given the subject any serious thought, he is led to consider those objects which he formerly pursued with avidity as altogether vain and delusive, and to devote the whole of his time and every mental energy, exclusively to the investigation of this now all-absorbing subject. When he finds that his conduct has been diametrically opposite to the pure morality of the gospel, and unhappily applies to himself the awful denunciations of Scripture, without receiving the consolations of its promises; the anticipation of that eternal misery, which he fancies to be his inevitable doom, continually fills his mind with gloomy apprehensions, and eventually sinks him into the most suffering state of insanity, from the over action of the brain in thinking on this subject.

W. A., a cheesemonger, about thirty-six years of age, is married, and has a family. About ten years ago he became much alarmed by the denunciations in the Bible against wilful sin; and the effect was so powerful, that he could not sleep at all for a fortnight. He then, being distracted, was sent to the workhouse, and from thence speedily removed to a private madhouse. Not finding any religious consolation, he determined upon making some sacrifice to obtain it. For this purpose, taking the words of Scripture in a literal sense, he attempted to pluck out his right eye. Self-injury was prevented, but he continued in agony, and generally on his knees, refusing every encouragement or consolation. After enduring this state four years, he was conveyed to the Asylum at Hanwell, where he became by degrees more composed, and he was, after some time, persuaded to attempt shoemaking.

This had a happy effect; he gradually recovered, and was discharged. He remained at home, and provided for his family one year and five months. Another attack then coming on, he was sent back to Hanwell, and remains there alternately sane and insane.

M. D., aged forty-two, has been insane some years. Erroneous views on religion are said to be the cause of the disease.

It appears, that some years ago she was living with a married cousin and her husband. She was in the habit of repeating to the husband the conversations which passed between her cousin and herself, especially when he had been the subject of them, and had been spoken of with opprobrium. In consequence of these communications, quarrel took place between the husband and wife, and they eventually separated. She became extremely sorry for her conduct when it was too late. She considered that she had been guilty of a great crime, and that no pardon from God would ever be shown to her for it; and to this hour she entertains the distressing and erroneous idea, that she has sinned the unpardonable sin against the Holy Ghost, and that eternal misery is her inevitable doom. She is generally in delicate health, and is kept as much employed as possible, to divert her mind from the gloomy thoughts which continually obtrude themselves upon her.

T. A., thirty years of age, had been insane one

year before admission. The disease came on gradually, from intense thought and anxiety on religious subjects. He was married, but had led rather a dissolute life, and, though not a drunkard, was in the habit of spending his time, and the money which ought to have supported his family, at the public-house. He became awakened to the true state in which he stood as a sinner before God; and over-looking all the promises of pardon contained in the gospel to those who truly repent, or imagining they could not apply to him, he became miserable. He saw nothing but condemnation before him, without one ray of hope. His sleep was gone,—the brain, overworked, lapsed into a state of great irritability, and insanity followed. In his hallucination he imagined that he was different from all other men, not only in the operations of his mind, but in the formation of his body; that he was without blood. Having requested, in vain, that he might be bled to prove it, he one day took an opportunity of seizing a knife, and with one blow he nearly severed the fore finger of the left hand. Though the operation convinced him of this error, others remained equally as absurd. His mind was always in such a state of perturbation that he could not for a long time compose himself sufficiently to settle to any employment. By degrees light at length dawned upon him; he began to perceive that though the threatenings of the Scriptures are most alarming to the impenitent, yet the hopes and consolations they contain to the

repenting sinner are equally powerful ; and with
this confiding view he was enabled to lay aside all
his unnecessary anxieties.   The overwrought action
of the brain had happily not produced diseased
organization ; he perfectly recovered, and returned
to his family, a better and a happier man than he
had ever been before.

The next primary moral cause which we shall
notice is Grief.   Females form by far the largest
proportion of this class.   The greater part of them
have become deranged from loss of their children.
After what we have already said, it will be unnecessary to point out the steps by which insanity,
from this cause, may also be traced to over-action
of the brain.   As in the preceding cases, irritation,
want of sleep, and subsequent inflammation, are the
general symptoms and consequences.

R. W., a female about forty-five years of age, has
been insane some time.   She lost two or three
children very suddenly, either from fever or small-
pox.   She was a most affectionate mother, and
became inconsolable for her loss.   At the time of
her admission, all the violence of her grief had
abated.   She seemed to have forgotten the particular circumstances of their death, and appeared
only conscious of their absence, without being able
to account for it.   She used constantly to walk
about the gallery and bed-rooms, looking behind
every door and into every corner, expecting to find
them ; and, if she could wander into the garden, or

about the premises in any direction, her only business was to seek for her children, and then return lamenting her disappointment. By degrees, she was induced to employ herself. She recovered her health, and ultimately got quite well, and was discharged about eighteen months after her admission.

S. T. had been insane two years when admitted. She was sitting with her husband at breakfast, and remarked to him, that she thought he appeared unwell; but he said, " No, he was much as usual." In a short time she left him, and went up stairs. She had scarcely gone out of the room, when she heard a sudden noise, as if something had fallen down ; she immediately ran down stairs, and found that her husband had fallen out of his chair on the ground, and was unable to rise. He spoke to her, and she ran to the next door, to send some one for medical assistance ; but when she returned, he was a corpse. In consequence of this sudden bereavement, she was left with four children entirely destitute. A subscription was raised on her behalf : but the effect of this sudden shock on the nervous system produced a depression of spirits so overwhelming, that she was incapable of attending to any thing : she could obtain no sleep, and was accustomed to walk her room, in an agony of grief, all the night long. Notwithstanding every kindness that could be shown to her, she became worse, and was ultimately removed to a public hospital, from which she was discharged as incurable. She at length died from pure exhaustion.

H. G., aged thirty-six, had only been insane three weeks when admitted. She was in a most distressing state of misery, arising from poverty and remorse. It appears that, some time ago, she was reduced to the most abject beggary, and unable to obtain food for herself and her little boy, who was about four or five years old. Under this pressure, she was induced to sell her child to a chimney-sweeper for a guinea. She had scarcely done the deed before she repented of it; and she set out to find the man, return the money, and reclaim her child. She soon became much excited, she wandered about all night in every direction, but could not hear any tidings of him. In addition to the painful feelings thus naturally produced, she had the mortification either of losing, or of being robbed of, the very guinea for which she sold him: this she considered a just punishment for the crime of which she had been guilty. She continued wandering about from place to place, going to all the chimney-sweepers she could hear of, and making every inquiry, but all in vain. Her child was never found again. The health of the body and powers of the mind, as might be supposed, at length sunk under the united effects of want and anxiety. She was picked up as a lunatic vagrant, and sent to the Asylum at Wakefield, where I left her unimproved, two years after her admission.—

In this instance, remorse was, probably, as much the cause of the insanity as grief.

The violence done to the natural affections, as recorded in the above cases, is not however the only mode in which grief brings on the disease. The following is a striking instance of its occurring from a purely moral feeling.

J. F. had been a porter eighteen years in one warehouse, and he possessed the confidence of his employer. There was a general order for all the inmates to return to the house by ten o'clock at night; this he disobeyed; and displeasing his master, a misunderstanding took place between them, which terminated in separation. The loss of his situation and of his master's confidence overwhelmed him with anguish; and though he entered into business with most favourable prospects, he was unable to attend to it, and did not succeed. This augmented his grief, and sleep was banished by constant watchfulness, accompanied with pain in the head. These symptoms increasing, he became insane, and was removed to an asylum. He has partially recovered, but has been subject to relapses ever since.

There are, however, one or two moral causes, the powerful effects of which upon the system are universally acknowledged, but by no means easy of explanation. How are we to account for the mode in which sudden joy or terror sometimes instantaneously destroys life, and sometimes as instantaneously brings on idiocy or insanity?

Several instances of death, produced by the sudden effects of Joy, are mentioned by Dr. Mason Good; and he also gives the particulars of a case which occurred to himself, in the person of a clergyman with whom he was intimate, but whose death was not so immediate.

This gentleman, who had consented to be nominated one of the executors of the will of an elderly person of considerable property, with whom he was acquainted, received a few years afterwards, and at a time when his own income was but limited, the unexpected news that the testator was dead, and had left him sole executor, together with the whole of his property, amounting to three thousand pounds a-year in landed estates. He arrived in London in great agitation, and on entering his own door dropped down in a fit of apoplexy, from which he never entirely recovered; for though he gained his mental and much of his corporeal faculties, his mind was shaken and rendered timid; and hemiplegia had so weakened his right side, that he was incapable of walking further than a few steps.

A melancholy instance of the sudden effect of terror happened a few years ago in the north of England. A lady had gone out to pay an evening visit, at which she was expected to stay late. The servants took advantage of the absence of the family to have a party at the house. The nurse-maid, in order to have enjoyment without being disturbed by a little girl who was entrusted to her care, and who would not remain in bed by herself, determined upon frightening her into being quiet. For this purpose she dressed up a figure, and placed it at the foot of the bed, and told the child if she moved or cried it would get her. In the course of the evening the mother's mind became so forcibly impressed that something was wrong at home, that she could not remain without going to ascertain if any thing extraordinary had occurred. She found all the servants dancing and in great glee; and on inquiring for her child, was told that she was in bed. She ran up stairs and found the figure at the foot of the bed, where it was placed by the servant, and her child with its eyes intently fixed upon it, but, to her inexpressible horror, quite dead.

A case occurred within my own observation, where insanity was the immediate consequence of fright. A woman was walking through the market of a town in Yorkshire with her husband, and seeing a crowd, she went to learn the occasion of it, when a large dancing bear, which a man was showing the public, suddenly turned round and fixed his fore paws upon her shoulders. She became dreadfully alarmed. She was got home as soon as possible; but the excitement was so great, that she could not sleep, nor could any thing persuade her but that the bear was every moment going to devour her. At the time I first saw her, which was some months after the occurrence, she was in the most pitiable state of distress, obstinately refusing all food, which she thought was only given to her to fatten her for the bear. She got no sleep, and was in great terror from hearing the noise of the *steam engine*, which was near the ward in which she was placed. She was removed into another, out of the sound, as she imagined, of the grumbling of the bear ; and she afterwards slept better. She was kept alive for nine months by food being forced into the stomach, but never without having to overcome all the resistance she could possibly make. In the end she became consumptive, and died.

In these, and similar cases, the immediate effect of the sudden shock upon the nervous system is to diminish the action of the heart ; and where death is the result, this action ceases entirely. When the shock is not so violent as to cause an entire stoppage, the heart gradually resumes its functions ; but the circumstances which caused the shock continue vividly impressed upon the mind, and produce excessive action in the brain ; and we find in these cases, after the first effect has subsided, the same watchfulness and excessive sanguiferous action in the brain, which accompany insanity when it arises from any other moral cause. The manner in which idiocy is brought on, is of more difficult explanation. It is probable that in these cases the brain sustains, from the sudden retreat of the blood, some physical injury, which is never afterwards recovered ; but after all our surmises, we must acknowledge **our** ignorance of the precise mode in which the senses act, so as to produce such powerful effects.

Mortified pride, disappointed love, jealousy, and, in fact, any other feelings which excite the brain to undue action, produce insanity as effectually as any of the moral causes of it which we have previously enumerated.   The following are some of the cases which have come under my *own* observation, where it has originated from these feelings :—

J. W. had been insane twelve months.   He was a young man about twenty-three years of age, whose connexions could not be considered as paupers, nor would he have become one had he not been rendered incapable of any employment by an attack of insanity.   He had been an apprentice to a retail shopkeeper in the country.   He had a fine person and pleasing manners, with a large share of self-esteem, combined also with much love of approbation.   He was altogether a very romantic person ; and having fallen in love with a young lady, he felt no doubt in his own mind that, as soon as his intentions were made known, he should be accepted. He was very pedantic in his manner ; and being anxious that all his proceedings should be conducted in the most correct manner, he proceeded very formally to make his proposals.   To his utter astonishment, they were not only rejected, but he was dismissed, to use his own expression, " with the most contemptuous scorn."   This was more than his offended pride could bear.   It was not the loss of the lady that affected him so much as the mode in which his offer had been received. It totally overcame him; he could get no rest night or day, and incurable insanity followed. At the time of his admission he had lost all the painful feelings which annoyed him on the first coming on of the disease, and he amused himself by imagining that he was some great man. He was very obliging, and for a long time assisted as a clerk in the office. He died of consumption about eleven years after his admission.

E. C., a female about thirty years of age: how long she has been insane is not exactly known. This case, like the preceding, was the consequence of offended pride. She was a fine young woman, but of ambitious views. She too, had become attached to a person in a more elevated situation of life than herself; and the mortification of being rejected, on account of the difference of rank, was a wound to her pride which she could not brook: she became incurably insane. Many years of mental suffering have not in the least tended to abate her self-esteem; and though she acts as a servant, in which capacity she lived before the attack, when unemployed in actual domestic duties, she never fails to display her pride, by assuming a very digni-fied carriage, and acting with the greatest *hauteur* towards all around her, especially if she has an opportunity of doing so before strangers. She is extremely fond of dress; but, in order to excite attention, will adorn herself even grotesquely, rather than not be thought singular. The gratification of these harmless passions appears to afford her much pleasure. She is in general very happy, but there is no hope of the disease ever being cured.

M. T., aged thirty, has been insane four months. Cause of the attack, disappointment in love. She formed an engagement with a young man, about six years ago; and he left her, after promising marriage. She says, that she has never been comfortable in her mind since, though she has worked regularly until within a few weeks. But she has shown evident symptoms of derangement : she neglected her business, and returned to her friends, saying, her state of mind would not permit her to work. About a week before her admission, she passed a whole night in the street, and she has since meditated self-destruction. Was discharged, cured, in eleven months.

E. S., aged thirty-seven, is married, and has been insane five years from jealousy of her husband. She has been a laundry-woman, was twelve months at St. Luke's, and afterwards went to visit her friends in Dorsetshire. She has a most violent antipathy to her husband, and no kindness or conciliation on his part at all softens it. He is very attentive, and brings her tea, and other little luxuries not provided in the house ; but all are ungraciously received, and sometimes she adds blows to her words. When she is employed, which, happily for herself as well as others, is generally the case, she is tranquil; but the slightest allusion to her husband is sufficient at once to throw her into a paroxysm of rage.

M. D., thirty years of age, had been insane only a few weeks. She had been brought up as a dress-maker, but unhappily had been seduced by an officer, to whom she was very much attached; after living with him for some time, he deserted her for another. Grief, mortified pride, and jea-lousy, all combined, produced a state of excitement which ultimately ended in insanity. She had sleep-less nights, the natural secretions were disordered, and violent mania was the consequence. It hap-pened unfortunately that my wife had so strong a resemblance to her rival, that nothing could per-suade her but that she was the identical person. In consequence of this similarity, whenever she went into her presence her rage knew no bounds. This irritation was avoided as much as possible by the patient being usually shut up in her own room before the former passed through the wards; but on one or two occasions, unfortunately, this precaution had been neglected, and the patient flew upon her with the savageness of a tiger, and literally pulled nearly all the clothes from her person before the nurses could rescue her from her grasp. On a subsequent occasion she accidentally found herself alone with her in an upper gallery, used only as a dormitory;

she disappeared on a sudden, when my wife instantly ran to the door, and had just time to get through it before she came up. When out of sight she had gone into one of the rooms to get a large leaden pot, with which she said she had intended to murder her. She was not violent against any one else, and would sometimes even beg of her, as she had got her lover from her, that she would be kind to him. She died of consumption in about two years.

Having considered those causes which act primarily upon the brain, whether physical or moral, let us now proceed to investigate those, which affect it by sympathy. It will be scarcely necessary to enter into any argument to prove, that the brain and nervous system sympathize with every other part of the body. Upon what other supposition could we account for the fact, that the irritation of teething, worms in the intestines, punctures in different parts of the body, will give rise to convulsions, which are universally allowed to be the consequences of disordered brain? The morbid action of the part primarily diseased, spreads itself along the whole chain of nerves, until it reaches the sensorium; irritation is caused there, and hence arise the convulsions. This irritation, however, when once produced, will not always cease on the discontinuance of the cause; and thus the convulsions frequently remain for some time after the primary cause of them has been removed. It is precisely in the same manner that diseases of the stomach, liver, lungs, intestines, &c.

so operate upon the brain as to produce insanity. A large class of patients from sympathetic causes, and by far the most easily cured, are those who have become insane from disorder of the chylopoietic viscera. A train of hypochondriacal symptoms usually exists in them for a length of time before they can be pronounced decidedly insane.

F. G., aged forty-one, has had repeated attacks of insanity. No cause for the disease coming on can be assigned but the disordered action of the chylopoietic viscera. He is an honest, sober, and hard-working man, an affectionate husband, and a kind father, except when suffering from this distressing malady. The attacks are usually preceded by his tongue becoming white and furred, his breath fœtid, digestion bad, with pain in the epigastric region, and bowels costive; he begins to be restless, complaining of some pain in the head; the eyes become red, and he imagines invisible spirits come to tell him of his wife's infidelity. It often requires very active purgatives to procure evacuation, and it is necessary to relieve the head by local bleeding and cold applications. As soon as these objects are accomplished, the symptoms gradually abate; and as no real moral cause exists to keep up the disordered action, it subsides altogether; but it is necessary to be extremely attentive to the state of the digestive organs, not only when he is recovering, but when he is in his best health; for if he allows the digestive organs to become disordered, an attack of insanity is as sure to follow, as quinsey does in those liable to that disease, when they have been exposed to severe cold.

It is often very difficult to determine whether the disease of the chylopoietic viscera has not in reality arisen from, instead of produced, diseased action of the brain ; as the stomach, intestines, &c. sympathize quite as much with the brain as the brain does with them. When, however, we are unable to find out any other cause for the mental alienation, and perceive that it ceases as soon as the secretions are restored to a healthy action, we have a right to conclude that the origin of the disease has been in the chylopoietic viscera.

We have many cases of insanity where the brain has apparently become affected by sympathy with diseased lungs. But as in the early stages of it, disease is rarely found to exist simultaneously in both the lungs and the brain, but rather appears to alternate from one to the other, our ignorance of the previous history of the patients, and the impossibility of finding out how long a disease of the lungs may have existed undiscovered, makes it most difficult for us to determine which of the two has first been attacked. In many cases this form of insanity seems to be combined with hereditary predisposition.

Many years ago I had a very interesting young woman under my care, a Moravian, who had been labouring under cerebral excitement for some little time, but by no means violent. No cause was assigned for the disease coming on. She had been educated, as persons of that sect generally are, with the strictest attention to all the moral virtues; and her whole conduct and demeanour, notwithstanding her insanity, were so engaging as to interest every one around her. She was not long before she began to improve mentally; but as the mind improved, it was evident some disease was going on in the chest. She began to have a cough, with a slight pain in her side. She had the usual remedies applied under such circumstances, which had the effect of diminishing the symptoms; but no sooner did these begin to subside, than the excitement again commenced in the cerebral organs. After a period these again abated; but as sanity returned, the pulmonary disorder came with it; and thus first one affection, and then the other, alternately predominated, until nature sank under the successive attacks.

J. J. had been insane about twelve months before his admission. He was a painter and glazier, and succeeded his father, who had died a short time before, leaving him a good business and some property. He no sooner got into possession of this, than he began to launch out into extravagant expenses, much beyond his means; and instead of being diligent to increase his income, so as to meet his enlarged expenditure, he neglected his business altogether, and finally became a bankrupt. This alteration in his circumstances, combined with intemperate habits, brought on insanity. A very considerable improvement took place in him mentally, after he had been confined about three months; and he employed himself at his business, and was about to be discharged, when he was seized with hœmoptysis. He recovered from this attack; but as the disease of the chest abated, the cerebral excitement was increased to a much greater degree than it had ever been before. Ultimately phthisis came on, and in the same degree as the diseased action of the lungs became violent, there was in general an abatement of the maniacal symptoms, though from the first attack of the pulmonary complaint, he could scarcely ever be said to be so sane as he had been immediately prior to its coming on.

Exposure to cold, which in most constitutions produces inflammation of the lungs, rheumatism, quinsey, &c. is not unfrequently the immediate cause of insanity in those who have a great predisposition to disease of the brain.

T. C., a labouring man, thirty-nine years of age, is reported to have been very maniacal for ten days. He had been washing sheep, and exposed to cold and wet, particularly in his lower and upper extremities, for some days prior to the attack. This appears to have been the immediate cause of its coming on; but it is stated that he had an uncle insane, and he had himself suffered a disappointment in not receiving some money which a relation had left him by will. He died exactly three months after admission. There was but little disease observable in the brain.   Half an ounce of serum was found in the ventricles, and the arachnoid was opaque.

W. F., a blacksmith, age twenty-eight, had been insane twelve months prior to admission.   He is reported to have had no symptom of the disease until he went into a cold bath about a week before he was attacked.   At the time of going in he was in a state of great perspiration.   It appears from his wife, that an alteration in his manner was perceived almost immediately after : he became low and desponding, his temper was naturally bad.   He recovered in about three months.

Much of the insanity amongst the agricultural labourers is to be traced to their exposure to cold, and to the vicissitudes of the weather, combined with their poverty and their indifferent diet.

Not only do we find that exposure to partial cold and checked perspiration are causes of insanity, but such a sympathy seems to exist between the brain and the skin, that in some individuals, when a cutaneous eruption has been repelled, a seton or an issue dried up, or an old ulcer healed too rapidly, the disease has been transferred to that organ, and has produced insanity in some cases, paralysis in others ; and as the brain suffers from the stoppage of an external discharge, so also is the same effect produced by the sudden suppression of the natural secretions and internal evacuations ; whether they be healthy and natural, as the menses and the milk, or unhealthy, as in hœmorrhage from the lungs, nose, piles, &c., or in diarrhœa.

R. H., aged twenty-four, had been for many years a nursery maid in a family of distinction. She was a young woman of exemplary character, and esteemed for her kindness and attention to the children. An alteration had been perceived in her conduct for eight or nine months before I saw her. She had become anxious and melancholy, without any apparent cause. Her former activity and diligence were succeeded by languor and irksomeness in every act. She complained to me that she seemed to have lost all mental feeling; the children on whom she used to doat, and a respectable young man, to whom she was shortly to have been married, after an engagement of some continuance, were now both disregarded by her, and she could not account for this; in fact, all natural affection seemed gone. She more especially lamented, that religion had lost its usual power to comfort her: all was changed. At this time she lived with a cottager, whose wife was a laundress, and had a family. On inquiry, I found that the catamenia, from what cause she was unable to explain, had not appeared for some time prior to the presence of these symptoms; the bowels were costive, and the liver torpid. After she had taken alteratives and emmenagogues, and used the hip bath for some time without effect, leeches to the labia pudenda relieved her on their first application.

The secretions afterwards took place in their natural course, and she got perfectly well. During the time when she was using the remedies, she was actively employed in walking to considerable distances, and took an interest in needle-work. She returned to her situation, and has since married the young man to whom she was engaged before her indisposition.

Women who have any predisposition to insanity, seem, both during pregnancy and immediately after delivery, more susceptible of its attacks than at any other periods. An inflammatory diathesis is, in fact, so commonly an attendant upon the state of gestation, that during some part of the time, in many cases, it is found necessary to abstract a few ounces of blood from the system. Now when the brain is the part attacked, and the disease is allowed to go on unchecked, insanity is very frequently the result.

M. N., about thirty-four years of age, became insane during pregnancy. No other cause could be assigned for the appearance of the disease coming on. She was in a state of great excitement when admitted, and continued so for two months, when she was confined. Very soon afterwards an alteration for the better took place ; the cerebral irritation gradually ceased. No untoward circumstances whatever occurred. She soon became interested in her child, and maternal feelings overpowered every other. She was discharged perfectly well within three months.

The following case was accompanied by distressing

melancholia ; but it disappeared as rapidly as the former after child-birth. The patient became insane about three months after pregnancy had taken place; but she was not sent to the Asylum until three months afterwards. She was then in a state of melancholia. She took no notice of any thing around her, and was perfectly mute. She was confined about two months after her admission. The pains of child-birth at once aroused her dormant feelings. The child was still-born ; but all the secretions coming on in the natural course, she quickly recovered. It appeared from her own statement that she had long been living in a state of concubinage with a man to whom she had borne several children ; but so deeply was she now impressed with the sinfulness of her conduct, that, though the man repeatedly came to her and urged her to return, no solicitation could prevail; she would not even see her children, unless she was first married. The man was very fond of her, (and they appear to have lived unmarried more from a thoughtlessness of the vice, than from any objection to marriage on his part,) and he readily consented. The banns were properly proclaimed in the parish church, the parties were married from the Asylum, and she returned with him to her former abode and family, cheerful and happy.

After delivery, insanity more frequently arises from the brain sympathizing with the uterus, from the stoppage of the lochia, or from its sympathizing with the breasts, from cold, or any other cause interrupting the secretion of the milk.

J. G., about thirty-five years of age, had been insane about six weeks when admitted. The disease came on four days after her confinement. She says, she awoke with an impression that the nurse had overlaid her child. A fever immediately ensued, the natural secretions ceased, she became sleepless, and insanity followed. She was in a very high state of mania when she arrived,—incessantly talking, mischievous, and destructive; tearing in pieces her clothes, bedding, and whatever came in her way. It was some months before any improvement took place. The bowels and other secretions were at length brought into their natural order, when she began to recover. In the course of a few weeks afterwards she was induced to work in the garden. From this time her recovery was very rapid. Her husband and friends came to see her, and she was much cheered by it, having only before seen them when she was incapable of appreciating the kindness of their visit. She was perfectly recovered and restored to her family in ten months.

M. A. B., a single woman, about twenty-four years of age, had an illegitimate child a few months before her admission. She is reported to have taken cold soon after her confinement; this was attended with fever, the flow of milk ceased, and insanity was the immediate consequence. Very little information could be obtained respecting her.

Her head was hot, and her bowels costive. She continued in a low, depressed state, refusing to occupy herself in any way for a considerable time. The natural secretions were disordered, and difficult of correction. It was not until fourteen months after her admission that she became interested in some new work, the spinning of twine, which had just been commenced in the ward where she was. This she was persuaded to attempt, and by degrees she employed herself in it many hours a day. The exercise of walking up and down the gallery, one hundred and eighty feet long, had a most beneficial effect. She soon began to improve in her general health, all the secretions became regular and healthy, and in a few months she was quite well.

E. S., aged fifty-seven, has been more or less insane twenty-four years. She says, she was first attacked after she had been confined about a week; she caught cold, when the milk, and other secretions, immediately ceased. She recollects being extremely violent, and getting out of bed without any clothes. She was sent to one of the public hospitals, and remained there some time. She recovered sufficiently to go into service for a short period, when she again became deranged, and has been alternately better and worse ever since. She has occasionally a maniacal paroxysm, but it lasts only a short time.

Where puerperal insanity has once occurred, whenever pregnancy takes place subsequently, the irritation very frequently reproduces the disease. We have had several cases of relapse under similar circumstances. This, however, may sometimes be prevented by carefully watching all the premonitory symptoms, and guarding against it.

H. S., aged twenty-five, the wife of a kind-hearted labouring man, was brought to bed of her second child in June, 1821 : about ten days afterwards she became insane. Her husband was unwilling that she should be sent to the Asylum, and she was kept at home for two months. She was then admitted as a patient into the institution at Wakefield; she was in a very emaciated state, with a quick and feeble pulse, bowels confined, wild and incoherent in her language, and the countenance showed that much diseased action was going on in the brain. The bowels were kept open by aperients, a blister was applied to the back of the neck, and the general health supported by nutritious diet. She was a little relieved by these means. On the fourth of October she had improved in her bodily health, and was also more rational. From this time until the ninth of November, little alteration took place mentally. She had then grown stouter in person, but was very little better in mind, and she complained of pain in the head: the bowels were confined. There had been no appearance of the catamenia since her confinement. Leeches were ordered to be applied to the temples. She took emmenagogues, and her bowels were kept regularly open. From this time she improved daily; she became quite rational, and was discharged cured about four months after her admission.

Soon after her next confinement, which took place in about two years, symptoms similar to those which preceded the former attack made their appearance; a sudden cessation of the secretions, quick pulse, hot and dry skin, with confusion of mind. She became much alarmed at these feelings, apprehending another attack. As she lived very near me, I had an opportunity of seeing her immediately. Similar remedies to those applied two years previously were again resorted to, and not only was the violence of the attack prevented, but its duration was so short, that at the end of the month she was quite well.

Insanity is also the result of fevers, whether they be of an inflammatory, or of a low, debilitating nature, in the first instance, by the too rapid circulation of the blood through the brain; and in the second, from the weakness left by the disease in that organ, which continues when the other parts of the body have recovered their healthy tone.

The great mischief arising in practice from confounding the delirium of fever with insanity, by which it is often succeeded, will make a few observations, to enable us to distinguish between the two, highly necessary.

In delirium from fever there is a total derangement of all the intellectual faculties. The powers of perception suffer no less than the reasoning and affective faculties; the language of the patient is confused, and generally an unintelligible mass of words without any definite meaning.

Now in insanity it never happens that all the intellectual faculties are at the same time disordered, except when the patient becomes delirious from fever, to which he is of course as liable as those who are sane. The insane possess a knowledge of the objects around them, and a power of reasoning, although incorrectly; whilst in delirium, volition, and even consciousness seem to be suspended. We may also be certain, that, when the disordered action of the brain has continued some time after the fever which caused it has ceased, and the pulse is natural, whatever else may be the symptoms, the patient is insane, and not delirious.

B. C., a female, twenty years of age, came over from Ireland with a family as a servant. She had not been long in England before she was taken ill with a fever, which continued for some time. No information could be obtained of the treatment; but we learnt that after the other symptoms of fever abated, the brain continued very much excited. She was in a high state of mania when admitted, and she continued very noisy, dirty, and destructive, notwithstanding every effort to relieve her, for six months; during the whole of this time her appetite was good, and she appeared but little affected by the disease, except that she grew thinner.

A trifling abatement was after this time observed to take place; she began to sleep a little in the night, which she had scarcely done previously. She was permitted to walk about without personal restraint, and became quite well at the end of ten months.

J. B., a tailor, twenty-six years of age, has been insane five weeks: the disease was brought on by fever. At the time of his admission he was labouring under great maniacal excitement; pulse quick, and head very hot. He says, he had drunk a considerable quantity of rum before the fever came on. Cooling applications to the head, and the usual remedies to restore the secretions to a healthy state, soon allayed the disease. He became rational in about fifteen days, and at the end of seven weeks was discharged cured.

Vice, in all her forms, tends to weaken the constitution, and, so far as the brain participates in the general debility, to produce insanity. But there is a vice, the secret and unsuspected indulgence of which seems, in addition to its weakening the general powers, to have a specific and direct tendency, in many constitutions at least, to operate upon the brain and nervous system. Would that I could take its melancholy victims with me in my daily rounds, and could point out to them the awful consequences, which they do but little suspect to be the result of its indulgence. I could show them those, gifted by nature with high talents, and fitted to be an ornament and a benefit to society, sunk into such a state of physical and moral degradation as wrings the heart to witness; and still preserving, with the last remnant of a mind gradually sinking into fatuity, the consciousness that their hopeless wretchedness is the just reward of their own misconduct. This painful subject is more fully discussed in a note at the end of the volume. Other details, not exactly suited to meet the eye of the general reader, will also be omitted in the text, and similarly inserted.

From the reports that we receive with our patients, inebriety appears to be a very frequent cause of sympathetic insanity. In every case of drunkenness a morbid action exists in the brain; this generally ceases, and the brain recovers its tone in a few hours; but there are some constitutions in which, if the stimulus be repeated for a few days in succession, the irritation and excitement of the brain continued after the cause has ceased, and the man becomes insane.

T. J. when admitted had been insane some years: it was his third attack. He was a butler in a gentleman's family, where he remained for nine successive years. His first attack was brought on by excessive drinking. He went into Wales to visit his friends, and whilst there he indulged too freely in the use of spirituous liquors, which produced a nervous irritability of the brain, disturbed and sleepless nights, and for a short period he was quite unconscious; he was sent to an Asylum, where he remained some time, and was discharged. Being out of a situation, and unable to obtain his former place, he gave way to despondency and grief, and, with a view to relieve his feelings, he again had recourse to spirituous liquors, which soon brought on another attack. From this he also recovered; but such is now the irritable state of his brain, that upon the least excess a return of the disease comes on; at other times he is perfectly rational and capable of performing a variety of duties in the establishment. He has lately learnt to make sweeping brushes.

R. W., eighteen years of age, had been insane about three months before admission. He was left an orphan when young, and placed under the care of a guardian. His father had left him a little property, but not sufficient to live upon without pursuing some business. After leaving school he was consequently bound apprentice to a brush-maker. He soon began to associate with the dissolute, and became intemperate. He was dissatisfied with his trade, and conscious of possessing some little property, was impatient of control. He ran away from his place. Some time after he thought he should like to become a shoemaker; the guardian placed him with one; but, as might be expected, he soon fell into his former vicious habits, and again left his employment. He next obtained a situation as waiter at a tavern, where he had constant opportunities of freely indulging his inclination to drink. This he did almost without restraint, until he brought on a very high state of mania. It is not known what remedies were used during the first three months of the attack, but he was in a state of the most furious mania when admitted; and notwithstanding every effort was made to subdue it, he continued in that state for eight months before it could be overcome. He afterwards got quite well, and has returned to his shoemaking.

But it is not in this immediate and direct way only that the intemperate use of fermented liquors brings on insanity. The free indulgence in the use of them, it is well known, produces venous congestion of the liver, and a disordered state of the chylopoietic viscera in general. In constitutions where there is a tendency to this disease, either from an hereditary taint, or from any other cause, this congestion and disordered viscera often occasion functional disorder in the brain, and will, if unchecked in such constitutions, engender insanity as certainly as it follows from the effects of drunkenness repeated day after day; and more especially is this the case if, whilst labouring under this disordered state of the digestive organs, any moral cause, even of a slight nature, should arise to produce much anxiety of mind.

Delirium tremens, which is the result of habitually drinking ardent spirits to excess, is, in many cases, the precursor of insanity.

The ultimate effects produced upon the nervous system from taking opium to excess, are very similar to those which arise from spirit drinking; but as this vice is one not generally committed by the lower orders, either in Yorkshire or Middlesex, but few cases occurring from this source have come under my observation.

It is well known that inanition is a cause of insanity. Where men have, from peculiar circumstances, been deprived of food for a long time, as is the case with sailors who have remained at sea for days or weeks together in an open boat, almost entirely without provisions, before death has released them from their sufferings, insanity has very frequently intervened.

But even where the deprivation of food has not been endured to such an extent, yet the gradual diminution of it causes such a general weakness in the constitution, in which the brain participates, that insanity is often the consequence. The cases, however, of this kind which have come under my observation, have been so combined with poverty and other distressing circumstances, that they can hardly be said to have arisen entirely from inanition; though better diet, aided by moral treatment, without any medicine, has very frequently restored them.

Gout, which has been classed by many authors as a cause of insanity, is of such rare occurrence amongst the poor, that very few cases from this source have fallen under my notice. We have not had one instance where, as far as we could ascertain, gout has been the cause of insanity; but I have no doubt that if it, or any other disease, be suddenly repelled, it will, in some constitutions, fly to the brain.

Dropsy is another disease, which my own experience would not lead me to assign as a cause of insanity. That dropsical affections have existed to a considerable extent amongst the patients, both at Wakefield and Hanwell, I cannot deny; but they have usually occurred amongst those who have long been previously insane, and have generally been the symptoms of a gradual breaking up of the constitution rather than the cause of the disease. They are generally soon after followed by death.

We have now enumerated most of the usual causes of insanity, and referring to our previous classification of them, it will be seen that such of them as affect the brain primarily, are either physical injuries, or an over-exertion of the whole, or of some part of it, produced by moral causes; whilst our second class comprises all those cases where the disease of the brain has been the result of its sympathy with some other diseased part of the body. But whatever may have been the cause, in a very large proportion of *post mortem* examinations of persons, who had been insane for some time previous to death, the appearances of the brain clearly indicate the existence of long continued inflammatory action, that is, of an unhealthy excess of blood; and omitting the consideration of cases of compression which we have already noticed, may not its progress be thus traced?   The brain, or more frequently some portion of it only at the commencement of the disease, being unduly exercised, or suffering from irritation, caused by sympathy with some other diseased part of the body, demands and receives an accelerated supply of blood ; this accelerated supply, unless the cause be removed, continues, the tone of the brain gradually becomes weakened, and a morbid structure eventually takes place, not only in the portion of it at first attacked, but by degrees in the whole mass, and in the membranes.   The effusion of serum in the ventricles, and under the membranes, is the consequence of this diseased accelerated action ; and it increases in quantity as the disease advances.   The fact that pain is frequently not felt in any part of the head is no objection to the theory, as on dissection it has been discovered that organic disease has existed to a very great extent, yet the patients had never complained of any pain ; nor does the circumstance that in mania, large bleedings have seldom produced much permanent relief, militate against it.   In all those cases where insanity has not arisen from direct physical injuries, the result of the excessive bleedings from the system is to weaken the strength of the patient, but not necessarily to remove the cause of the diseased action.   If that be purely moral, of course this will be unaffected by the bleeding, and will still continue to produce an over-exertion of the brain, or of some part of it; and although the general volume of the blood will be diminished, yet the brain will receive an undue share of that which remains in the system, and the delusion, which is the result of this diseased action, will continue. If the cause of the disease be sympathy, the bleeding will be of use or not, according as it affects the disease of the part with which the brain sympathizes; but this subject will be considered more fully in the chapter on Treatment.

CHAPTER IV.

In the first chapter we have entered so fully into a description of insanity, that we have, in a great measure, anticipated the subject of the present one, at least as far as regards its general outline. Its various modifications are so numerous, that it would be quite impossible, in the limits to which we propose to extend this work, to give an account of each.

As utility is the principal object in view, it will be only necessary, then, to state those modes which are really important, and of the most frequent occurrence.

The misery which would be prevented, were the premonitory symptoms of its approach but generally known and carefully attended to, will amply justify our extending our inquiries to these symptoms.

When organic lesion of the brain exists, one of the first symptoms that is observed, is, that the intellectual faculties gradually become confused, the senses appear benumbed, there is embarrassment in speaking, and a general difficulty of articulation, as if the tongue had suffered a slight paralysis. In this stage the patient when roused will be able to give rational answers to questions of the kind that are usually put to him.

As the organic disease increases, we find a torpor in the limbs, and a gradual indisposition to any muscular exertion. The circulation becomes languid; there is a great congestion of the vessels of the extremities, particularly of the feet and legs, which are cold, purple, and often œdematous. A gradual emaciation of the system takes place, until at last death terminates the automatic existence.

When insanity arises from slow, spontaneous, inflammatory action of the brain, or its membranes, it is often, though not always, preceded by severe and continued pain in some part of the encephalon, which every mental exertion tends to increase; a variety of ideas seem to float across the mind without making the slightest permanent impression; there exists a consciousness, that the mind is wandering without a power of controlling its operations. Sometimes the senses become extremely acute, that of hearing in particular. When this spontaneous inflammatory action has proceeded so far as to cause insanity, the symptoms are the same as when the insanity has arisen from diseased action, produced by moral causes, which we shall notice immediately.

Intense abstraction of mind may be considered as the first alteration that is observable in the great majority of patients who become insane from moral causes.   The ordinary duties of life are either altogether neglected, or only performed upon the pressing solicitation of friends.   After this state has continued for a short time, it becomes necessary, if we wish to arrest the attention of the patient, to speak to him loudly and repeatedly; and when at last he seems conscious of what is said, he appears as if just aroused from a dream, and relapses into the same state of forgetfulness, as soon as the sound of the voice has ceased to vibrate in his ears; his whole air and manner evidently indicate that the inner man is dwelling upon a subject far different from that about which he is being addressed.   The general desire to please no longer influences the character, and the dejected looks, and the forlorn dress, sufficiently proclaim that the mind is entirely absorbed in its own contemplations.

This is the period when the alarm of friends ought to excite them to the most active measures; this is the time when the advice of a physician is truly desirable.   There is now an opportunity of resorting with success to measures, which will prevent the coming on of a malady, the treatment of which is at all times difficult, and which, if neglected at the commencement, is attended with circumstances the most painful to the patients and to their friends, and too frequently sinks the unhappy sufferers into a state of hopeless wretchedness, from which no remedies whatever seem able to release them. I cannot refrain from mentioning a case which fell under my own observation, and which will exemplify, in a striking manner, the consequences of neglect on the one hand, and of timely attention on the other.

Sarah C., aged twenty-eight, married, and has several children, was admitted into the Asylum at Wakefield in August 1824. She had been insane about five months. She had an aunt insane; but neither her father nor mother had been so. The attack came on from great anxiety, in consequence of one of her children having been lamed. Her husband and friends were unwilling to send her away, until, in a fit of despondency, she cut her throat very severely, and lost a great quantity of blood. After her admission, no medical remedies were required, except purgatives on the bowels becoming costive, and the application of a few leeches to the temples in October, in consequence of pain in the head. She gradually recovered, and was discharged December 10th. She continued quite well until July 1830, when she became abstracted, was seized with continued pain in the head, had restless nights, and said she felt much as she had done at the commencement of the former attack. She was greatly depressed in spirits, and alarmed at another coming on. The digestive organs were much disordered: head hot: pulse quick. I ordered twelve leeches to be applied to the temples, her head to be shaved, and kept constantly cool by thin cloths dipped in cold water, and her feet warm by the pediluvium. She took calomel and ext. colocynth as a brisk purgative. Her head was soon very much relieved; and after taking rhubarb, soda, and ginger, in small doses three times a day, for about a fortnight, she recovered both her health and spirits, and did not exhibit the slightest appearance of derangement. As no moral cause existed at home to keep up the excitement, I did not think it necessary to remove her, and she continued there during the whole period of the attack. This patient's life was nearly falling a sacrifice to neglect in the first instance; in the latter, timely attention entirely warded off the attack.

The silent abstraction most frequently arises from depressing causes. The symptoms of insanity produced by joy and unexpected success assume a different character. Under these circumstances, the alteration, which displays itself in the increased quickness and vivacity of the demeanour, the continued talking, and extravagant expressions of hope, is as indicative of an unhealthy action of the brain and nervous system, and requires to be as carefully watched on its very first appearance, as the depressing symptom of abstraction which we have just described. It must not be supposed that in order to make precaution necessary, incoherence must exist; or that the mind when called into action should be incapable of displaying its usual powers. These are amongst the last and severest consequences of an unhealthy action in the brain, which may exist without producing them for a considerable period; but as every prudent man, when he feels a pain in his chest, and a teasing cough, attended with fever, indicating an inflammatory action going on in his lungs, does not wait until the expectoration of pus has taken place, to denote that the disease has already reached the state of phthisis, before he sends for his physician ; so ought we to consider the premonitory symptoms we have mentioned, as the evidence of a diseased action of the brain having commenced, of which insanity is the end. And as we should look upon this even with more horror than we should upon consumption, so ought we still more carefully to use every possible expedient to prevent its approach. I know an instance where a man became insane from a sudden access of prosperity ; but no notice was taken of his altered conduct until he ordered a carriage and four to go to London to pay off the national debt. His friends then saw the necessity of placing him under medical care. It was too late; the disease had been allowed from neglect to gain a hold which was never recovered.

When insanity arises from the brain sympathizing with the chylopoietic viscera, the premonitory symptoms are dyspepsia combined with hypochondriasis, of which it is unnecessary to give a particular account. After the unhealthy action of the brain has proceeded to such an extent as to produce insanity, its symptoms, from whatever cause it may primarily have arisen, depend very much upon the natural character of the patient, except in the case of organic lesion of the brain, which we have mentioned already.   One of the most frequent modes in which these mental aberrations exhibit themselves, is by inducing a constant feeling of suspicion.   The patient continually fancies that every one is combining against his happiness; his most intimate friends and connexions, probably from being more immediately in contact with him, are the most frequently suspected, and are the subjects of his greatest aversion.   In these, as in all other instances of mental delusion, every attempt to convince the patients by reasoning of the extravagance of their notions, is worse than useless.

T. P., about sixty years of age, a short, fat man, with a red face, indicative of having been a hard drinker, came into the Asylum after having been insane only a few weeks.   The symptom first noticed was his altered manner to his wife, with whom he had formerly lived very happily, but whom he suspected of having determined to take away his life.   He was convinced she intended to poison him by mixing arsenic with the sugar which he put into his tea.   Upon no other subject did he appear the least irrational; but this delusion so haunted him, that he could settle to no business. He was continually moving about from one place to another, drinking considerable quantities of brandy and water at the same time.   It was necessary, at length, to send him to the Asylum.   The abstaining from spirits, and leading a temperate life, made a considerable improvement in him; but he still retains the notion that his wife intends to poison him.

Religious delusions, as will be readily anticipated from what has before been said on the effects of over-anxiety on this subject, are another very common symptom of insanity.   The whole topic of the patient's thoughts and conversation, is the eternal perdition that he feels assured inevitably awaits him.   This excessive anxiety about religious subjects is often found amongst those who have led the most virtuous and moral lives.   The same cautious feeling which produces such distressing fears for the future, has, when not over-excited, been previously the means of preserving them from falling into gross vices.   Many patients, particularly females, imagine that they are bewitched.

Mary W., aged forty-three, a remarkably fine woman, with very soft and pleasing manners, but of abandoned character, had been insane several years when admitted.   The only symptom of derangement she ever exhibited, was that of imagining she was beset with witches.   When at home, and occupied with her domestic concerns, she was quiet and industrious; but at other times she would go about the house with a lighted candle, threatening to burn it down.   I have frequently known her get up in the most violent agitation, go into the passage, and fight the witches, with whom she was continually

holding long conversations; but her principal intercourse with them was in the night. It seldom,
indeed, happened that she had not a violent complaint to make in the morning of the ill treatment
she had been receiving from them. They had
pinched and bruised her all over, and would allow
her to get no rest. The nurse used to report that
she often heard her fighting with them the greater
part of the night. She remained several years in
the Asylum, and, with the exception of her libidinous manners, conducted herself remarkably well.
She was very industrious, good tempered, and
obliging; but to the end of her life she retained the
notion that she was always under the influence of
witchcraft.

S. W., about thirty years of age, has been insane
for four years. This patient has no other symptom
of the disease but her peculiar notion of witchcraft.
She considers that she is under the influence of
three witches, one of blood, one of spirits, and
another of death, and that each takes possession of
her in turn. She is sometimes filled with the blood
of other people, her own being first abstracted. If
a patient in the ward, or one whom she has known
in any other part of the house, dies, she imagines
the spirit witch transposes the body of the dead
patient into her, and she suffers exceedingly from it.
Nothing can persuade her but the witch of death
frequently comes to her and stops the action of her
heart for a season, and then suddenly departs.

Another imagines that witches have power to throw gas upon her, so that she is almost suffocated with it.   She says, the first feeling she had of the kind, was on one evening when she was looking at herself in a glass, she suddenly saw something which she could not comprehend, and became dizzy.   She afterwards found it was high witchcraft, and that, besides throwing gas, the witches have the power of putting electricity into every part of her body.   She says, she is always glad of employment, for that they then keep most away from her.   The result, which her experience has taught her, that the mental delusion is the least powerful during the time of active employment, is not, as we shall have occasion to observe, confined to the cases where witchcraft is the subject of it.

It ought to be mentioned, that very few of the cases admitted into public institutions, where the disease has arisen from erroneous notions of suspicion or witchcraft, are entirely cured; and I attribute it to the following cause: the diseased action of the brain comes on so slowly, and the consequences of it are apparently so little injurious, either to the patient himself or to society, that it is permitted to go on unattended to, until it has existed for a very long period, and become a habit of the constitution, until, in fact, the notions interfere with the regular duties of life, and prevent the patient's having any intercourse with society.

Another very curious and frequent effect produced in the mind by insanity, is the hypochondriacal supposition of the existence of venereal
diseases. So strong is this delusion, that in one
instance, although there was no possibility of the
disease having existed, the patient fancied she had
been infected by it in some unaccountable mode,
and could not rest satisfied until put under a course
of what she imagined to be mercurial medicines.
After having taken these for a time, though nothing
more than pills made of bread-crumbs, the patient,
from the expectation that they were to produce
salivation, spat such a quantity of saliva as to require
a vessel constantly by her side for that purpose.
After this had continued for some time, she imagined that the medicine had produced its effect;
she discontinued the bread pills, and the excessive
action of the salivary glands ceased.

Another very frequent symptom of insanity is
the patients' entertaining very high notions of their
own consequence and ability. It would be an end-
less and useless task to give the history of all the
emperors, kings, queens, and nobles that we have
had in our *pauper* establishment; even Omnipotence
itself has not wanted a representative.

It has been stated in a former part of this work,
that when there has been an hereditary liability to
insanity, it is very apt to recur precisely in the same
manner from one generation to another; and that
this particularly happens in the case of suicide;

but not only does a tendency to suicide exhibit itself where there has been any hereditary predisposition to that particular form of the disease, but it is unfortunately a very general, and in many cases the only symptom of insanity, where there is no hereditary tendency to it.

Some persons are constitutionally so depressed and melancholy in their dispositions, that as the mode in which insanity exhibits itself depends very much on the natural character, the unhealthy action of the brain, occasioned only by some trifling circumstance, which to persons of another temperament would almost pass unheeded, in them increases the feelings of gloom and despondency to such an extent as to lead them to the commission of suicide. This is only, however, a symptom of insanity, and may reasonably be expected to be removed as speedily as most other forms of the disease. The consequences of it are so direful, that the most early and unceasing watchfulness is absolutely requisite.

Patients having this propensity, will have their periods of convalescence and of exacerbation precisely in the same manner as those, whose insanity assumes any other form, have their lucid intervals and paroxysms. I have known them remain for weeks together without the slightest disposition to injure themselves. In fact, in these patients, as well as in those who are liable to fits of rage and mischief, the particular propensity seems entirely to disappear for a season, during which personal

restraint is unnecessary. By far the greater proportion of patients of this class, who have been
admitted into the institutions at Hanwell and Wakefield, have been necessarily those in whom the
determination to destroy themselves has been pre-
meditated, and not the result of a sudden impulse.
The greater part of these consist of individuals of a
melancholy temperament, who have become insane
solely from hereditary predisposition, without any
other assignable cause.

It would be of very little practical utility to
enumerate those moral causes which, operating upon
a gloomy disposition, excite this painful propensity.
It sometimes arises from fear of disgrace or punishment ; and in this establishment some of the patients,
with unaccountable inconsistency, have been driven
to attempt the desperate act, from a conviction that
they were doomed to the severest everlasting punishment, the actual suffering of which, to their diseased
imagination, seemed more tolerable than its mere
anticipation.

The retiring from the pursuits of an active and
busy life has been stated as producing that feeling
of *ennui,* which has led to self-destruction ; but in a
pauper establishment, no patients of this description
are ever found ; nor do I recollect one case of this
kind in private practice, where there has not previously been such a habit of drinking, as might be
supposed to lead to organic disease ; and in these
cases the mode which has usually been adopted for

the destruction of life, has been by taking a large quantity of laudanum. I have not seen any of those cases of indirect suicide, or of the destruction of others, that the patients themselves might be punished with death,—stated by some authors to have proceeded from the patients imagining, that by the commission of this crime they should instantaneously secure to themselves eternal happiness; although I have no doubt of their existence.

Many cases of suicide, in those who have a natural predisposition to it, arise from the brain sympathizing with the liver; nor can this be a matter of surprise to any one, who has felt the depression of spirits incident to a disease of that organ. So many cases have occurred from this cause, that many writers, from not finding, on subsequent dissection, any organic lesion of the brain, have referred it to diseased viscera only. But as we find that the insanity ceases when the liver is restored to health, there is no reason for supposing that the insanity is, in these instances, any other than a disease of the brain.

J. C., about fifty years of age, has been insane about two years. He had formerly been in respectable circumstances, and occupied as a writer in an office. He is reported to have made several attempts on his life. Has been in the habit of drinking spirits very freely, and has a disease of the liver, which appears of some standing. At the time of his admission he was in a most emaciated state; his

legs scarcely able to support him.   His face and
body also were covered with an eruption ; tongue
furred ; his stools very dark : he was much depressed, and always moaning most piteously ; complained of heat and numbness in the head, and pain
in all his limbs.   Leeches and cold lotions were
applied to his head, his bowels opened by calomel
and colocynth, and he went into the warm bath
every other day.   He was much relieved by these
means.   He still continued, however, to moan as
before.   His tongue remained furred, and stools
unhealthy.   He took pil. hydrargyri gr. v. alter.
nocte for some time.   These were then left off
awhile ; no improvement taking place, he began the
pills again, and has continued them now for two
months with evident advantage.   His tongue has
become clean ; he is less depressed ; he is stronger,
and gaining flesh ; the biliary secretions are much
improved.   He now is occupied in the office ; and
every day, as the action of the liver seems to improve, his mind makes a corresponding advance.

It has before been observed that phthisis and
insanity alternate with each other ; and it does not
unfrequently happen that this peculiar symptom of
insanity, the tendency to suicide, has come on in
the very last stage of consumption. Many, who have
rushed unbidden into the presence of their Maker,
would, in the ordinary course of the disease, in a few
days have been released from their sufferings.

I had a patient in Hull, many years ago, who

was suffering in the very last stage of phthisis, and who could not apparently have lived many days. During the absence of his wife, who had left him for a short time, he cut his throat; and on her return she found him quite dead, leaning over the back of his chair, with a large pool of blood near him. She thought it had arisen from the lungs, as he had occasionally had hœmoptysis, until she made the melancholy discovery, that it was the result of his own act.

A singular expression of countenance, especially in the eye, has been noticed by many authors, as an unvarying attendant on a disposition to suicide. This, as well as the fœtor before described, certainly exists in a great many cases. Indeed, when powerful feelings or passions are in active operation, in the insane or in the sane, they draw the muscles of the face into particular forms; and if they continue for a length of time to be greatly predominant, they impress upon the countenance an appearance indicative of the character. This is felt and acted upon unconsciously in the common intercourse of life. A good countenance is a letter of recommendation; and we have, in spite of ourselves, an unfavourable feeling towards a stranger, where this is absent. Now in the generality of suicidal cases, the desponding feelings are in constant and active operation; hence there is usually a melancholy and gloomy expression of countenance. This arises from   no   mysterious   cause   peculiar   to insanity, but is perfectly intelligible on common physiognomical principles ; but there are numerous instances where the most experienced physician would be unable to detect, by inspection only, the slightest mark of either a disposition to suicide or insanity.   The absence of this expression must not, therefore, induce us to suppose, that this disposition does not exist.

The mode of self-destruction usually attempted by the patients, who have been brought into the Asylum at Wakefield and Hanwell, has been by hanging.   In some cases, so determined have they been to destroy themselves, that, even after admission, they have made the attempt in situations where the only point of suspension has been so low as to compel them to sit or kneel down, in order to accomplish their purpose ; and had they not been discovered by the keepers, in all probability they would have succeeded.

The particular mode by which suicides are desirous of accomplishing their purpose, appears to be a matter of much thought and consideration ; and after the plan is once settled, they seem to neglect all other means of self-destruction which may offer themselves, until they have an opportunity of perpetrating it in that particular way. An old man, upwards of seventy years of age, who had a market-garden near to the Asylum at Wakefield, came to consult me as to the best mode of destroying himself, as he had made up his mind not to live any longer.   He said he had thought of hanging himself, if I could not recommend an easier death. I talked to him for some time upon the heinousness of the crime he contemplated, and endeavoured to show him, too, that hanging was a most horrible death, from the suffocation that must be felt; but apparently with little success. Finding, however, that the chylopoietic viscera were a good deal disordered, I prescribed for him, and sent to inform his wife that he ought never to be left alone. The medicine had the effect of restoring the secretions to a healthy action, and he got better. I heard no more of him for some time, when I was at length informed that he was discovered dead in a little shed in his garden, where he used to keep his tools. But so fixed was the mode in his mind by which he was determined to accomplish his death, that, though the place was so low he could not even stand upright in it, and he had not a rope or even a string with which he could suspend himself, he contrived it by getting a willow twig and making it into a noose, which he fastened to one of the rafters. He stooped to put his head through it, and then pushing his feet from under him, suspended himself until he died. Now if he had not made up his mind to destroy himself in this particular way, he might have accomplished it with much greater ease by drowning himself in the pond in his garden, or by cutting his throat with his garden knife, which he always had about him; but neither of these was the mode he previously intended.

It may be practically useful to all who have the immediate care of suicidal patients, to bear this in mind ; and if they can find out that any particular plan is contemplated, they ought to be especially careful to remove the means of accomplishing it out of their reach, and to prevent their having an opportunity of carrying their particular plan into execution.

I had a patient some years ago who had attempted to hang himself, and was still bent upon doing it when he was admitted.   He eventually got well. He told me that for a considerable time after his admission he was constantly seeking for an opportunity of doing it, but was so closely watched that he could not succeed.   At the very same time this man was constantly employed as a carpenter with edged tools ; but self-destruction by those means he had never contemplated.

We have had an instance where a woman took a sheet from the bed, fastened one end of it round one of the foot-posts, and afterwards bringing the other end over the bed, then made a noose, into which she put her head, and sitting down, attempted, though ineffectually, to strangle herself.   Indeed, where the determination to effect their purpose is very strong, the arts which the patients resort to are scarcely to be credited by any but those who have witnessed them.

A female had made repeated attempts, during her residence in the Asylum at Wakefield, to hang herself, but had been so watched that she had not succeeded. One evening the servant, on going to remove all her clothes out of her bed-room, which is the regular practice, thought she saw something bright on the top of her chemise; upon examination, this was found to be a pin. She had contrived, just before bed-time, to take off her garter; and knowing that her pockets as well as her clothes would all be removed, she contrived to pin it within her chemise, so high up that it would not reach below the bottom of it. Very providentially, the brightness of the metal discovered it, and she was again prevented from accomplishing her purpose. By degrees the propensity wore off, and after a residence of eighteen years in the Asylum, I found her, a few months ago, living, though upwards of eighty years of age, in a comparatively tranquil state, waiting her removal in the ordinary course of nature.

After finding that they are so unceasingly watched, and so carefully secured, that they have no opportunity of executing their design, they will assume a most cheerful manner for days and weeks together, in order to lull suspicion; and when a favourable opportunity offers itself, it is never neglected.

A man who had long been in a state of despondency, and had made many attempts to hang himself, but had always been prevented, very suddenly appeared much better. He became apparently cheerful, and being desirous of employment, was sent

out with a large party into the hay-field. He continued in this, and other out-door occupations, for
some time, gradually improving. One evening, on
returning from the field, when the rest of the party
went in to tea, (which they were allowed when hay-
making,) he told the farming man that he did not
feel thirsty, and as it was very warm, he would
rather remain at the door. He was left there. A
short time afterwards his keeper came down to
inquire for him, and being told where he had been
left, immediately exclaimed, " Then he has hung
himself!" It was also singularly impressed upon his
mind, that it was in one particular out-house that
he had done it: there he went, and found him suspended and dead as he expected.

The principal symptoms to be noted of this fatal
tendency are general despondency and great abstraction, very frequently arising from the mind
contemplating how the purpose can be most securely
accomplished. After a time, if no opportunity has
offered to make the attempt, an affected cheerfulness
is sometimes put on in the presence of others; but
upon careful watching this will be seen only to exist
in company, and when alone the same gesticulations
and desponding expressions are exhibited as before.

It rarely happens that attempts at suicide are
made in the presence of others; but one of the
female patients who was under my care, would,
if she was at liberty for a minute, even though
the nurse was in the room with her, tie either her

handkerchief or her apron-strings tight about her throat, for the purpose of choking herself.

Suicides appear sometimes to take place from a sudden impulse, where no disposition to self-destruction has been previously shown or suspected. A young woman, about twenty years of age, who had been insane but a short time, and appeared to be recovering, after having assisted the nurse to whitewash and clean the ward, was sitting in the evening at tea with her and several other patients. She took the opportunity of the nurse going to a cupboard for some sugar, to seize a knife with which the nurse had just cut some bread; and in the presence of the whole party, in an instant, before her hand could be arrested, cut her throat in so dreadful a manner that she died almost immediately.

Amongst other symptoms usually noticed by writers on the subject, is the change that very often is observed to take place both in the passions and propensities. It frequently happens in cases of insanity, that persons of an amiable and benevolent temper become, when insane, highly mischievous and violent; and modest and reserved females give utterance to language the most opposite to that which might have been expected from their previous habits.

A patient in the Asylum at Wakefield, the wife of a labourer, a kind-hearted and clever woman, was afflicted with such a propensity to destroy, that she was almost constantly obliged to be kept in confinement; and when at liberty, she could not resist the pleasure of breaking any thing she met with. In one instance she saw some tea-cups on a table, and for some time walked backwards and forwards, and checked the inclination; but eventually the temptation proved too strong, and she swept them at once on the floor. She afterwards regretted the circumstance; but the impulse was too powerful to be resisted. Numbers of similar cases, and of instances of change in the conversation and demeanour of virtuous females, might, if necessary, be enumerated; but it will be more to the purpose to try to explain the causes on rational principles.

In a state of sanity the various feelings and propensities are kept under control, partly by their mutual inflence upon each other, partly from moral causes, and partly from the restraints imposed by society. And where careful education and religious feeling have rendered their due regulation habitual, strong propensities may exist unknown and unsuspected, except by the individual. Now insanity does not create any new class of feelings or propensities. It is, I am aware, a very common opinion, that persons, in consequence of their becoming insane, acquire a new set of faculties, and especially that they become endowed with a great share of cunning. This is quite an error. There is no doubt but that this faculty may be often found very powerfully and actively developed amongst them; but where this is the case, it must have existed in the character previously to the disease coming on. A great number of the patients in public asylums, so far from being particularly cunning, possess no fraudulent dexterity of any kind. The mode in which insanity acts, is to cause an alteration in the mental manifestations and in the conduct, by exciting some to undue exercise, and not permitting others to have their proper influence. Where the passions are thus over-excited, and the controlling feelings are not in sufficient activity, we have necessarily the results previously mentioned; nor ought they to excite in us any surprise, even when observed in the most virtuous and amiable.

Another circumstance of a very painful character is frequently attendant upon insanity, and, as far as I know, no attempt has yet been made to account for it. I am referring to the change which takes place in the affections towards those to whom the patients have formerly been the most attached. This change generally takes place in those cases where the patients themselves are quite unconscious of the existence of any disease, and where it has come on by slow degrees, and is only very partial in its effects. This unconsciousness, I should observe by the way, is by no means universal in insanity; in many cases the patients themselves are perfectly aware that something is wrong.

When the alteration produced by the insanity has by little and little at length become so marked that even the most affectionate feelings can no

longer be blind to the painful reality of its existence, those whom the patient has been in the habit
of controlling, are obliged, for the safety of himself
and others, to apply not only moral but bodily
restraint, and to remove him from his home.   Not
being conscious of the necessity of such measures,
they appear to him harsh and unjust, and he thinks
that they emanate from a change having gradually
taken place in the feelings of those about him ; and
he is ready at once to exclaim, " You have ceased
to love me !"   As a proof that these feelings of
estrangement are thus produced, it is to be observed
that they seldom extend to those individuals of the
family who have been at a distance, or who are not
associated in the mind as having been accessory to
the restraint, first in trifling domestic matters, and
subsequently in removal from home, and confinement.   I think it may generally be taken for
granted, that though every other symptom of the
disease may appear to be removed, yet, so long as
this feeling of dislike continues towards those formerly loved, and who have really acted in an
affectionate manner, throughout all the trying scene,
to the unfortunate patient, that some lingering trace
of diseased action still continues, and the complaint
may be expected to return.

In cases where the patient is suddenly attacked
with mania, and his immediate removal from home
is necessary when he is hardly conscious of it, this
feeling does not exist.

The bodily symptoms, which occur so frequently in insanity as really to deserve to be considered as characteristics of the disease, are very few. The unhealthy action in the brain and its membranes is visible, rather from the alteration in the mental manifestations, than from any uniform corporeal change. In the early stages it is usually marked by irregularity of the secretions, yet it often happens, even in this stage, that, after it has continued for a short time, no alteration whatever takes place in the pulse, and all the secretions appear to be healthy. This is particularly the case where the symptoms denote only a small portion of the brain to be diseased, and where this disease has come on very gradually, the nervous system seeming to accommodate itself to the change, without being so irritated as to disturb the functions of the other parts of the body. And when the derangement has become chronic, it is a well-known fact, that many of the patients, for years together, enjoy excellent bodily health, and exhibit no marks of disease except mental delusions. It is probably this circumstance, which has led to the erroneous notion that medicine is of no use in all cases of insanity. It is singular that this uniformly good bodily health is rarely found, except in those cases where the hallucinations of the patient are confined to one subject.

Where the unhealthy action of the brain and nervous system has been so great as to produce deranged manifestation in the faculties generally, considerable bodily weakness and disease, of some kind or other, uniformly exists. The first thing which we ought to examine is the state of the head: it is there that we usually find a marked change. With very few exceptions, a considerable increase of temperature will be found in it, and it is often much hotter than other parts of the body, which are even covered with the clothes : when this is the case, the pulse is generally found quick,—but this increased temperature of the head sometimes exists, even to a great degree, without that being the case ; and when the heat is not very considerable, no variation whatever is usually to be found in the pulse : and this rule holds good whether the case be recent or of long standing.

S. M. has been insane and confined for many years,—in general very violent ; has been at Hanwell only eleven months and a half. She had not been long in the asylum before she became interested with the work that was going on in the garden, and requested to be employed. She continued working very quietly for six months. She afterwards thought she should like to learn brushmaking : this she also went on with very steadily for five weeks. She then became somewhat unsteady, rambling out of the workshop, and was soon irritated. It was found necessary to leave her in the ward, and not to permit her to go to work : she was offended and much excited. I suspected that some increased action of the brain was existing, either primarily from mental irritation, or from sympathy with the chylopoietic viscera; she was therefore carefully examined; her tongue was found much furred, her head extremely hot, and the pulse one hundred,—the usual range of it being, as I find from the notes kept of her case, about eighty. The stomach and bowels were immediately attended to, but no alteration having taken place, her head was ordered to be shaved, and cold applications used. This order occasioned the most violent excitement, as indeed did every other which was contrary to her own inclinations; but it was accomplished. The following day the head was cool, the pulse seventy, and the paroxysm subsided.

J. L., about thirty years of age, reported to have been insane but a short time. The tongue coated with a white fur, bowels costive, head hot. Complains of pain in the upper part of it. Pulse eighty-six and full. He took an emetic, and afterwards the diuretic drops, every four hours; the head was shaved, and cold applications used; in three days the pulse was reduced to sixty, and he was better in every respect.

W. P., aged twenty-one, has been insane about six months. He says it came on in consequence of going to a chapel to ridicule the preacher: but during the time he was there his conscience became so alarmed, that, his mother says, when he returned home he was in the greatest agitation, he got no sleep, and eventually became insane. On his admission, his head was very hot, pulse eighty-six, tongue dry, bowels costive. Head being shaved, cold applications used, and the bowels and secretions attended to, he was a little better for three days. Without any apparent cause, a more maniacal state came on, the pulse rising to one hundred, in which state he has continued for two days.

The two following cases are of long standing.

P. T. has been insane for several years. She has had repeated attacks, and been dismissed and re-admitted several times. She had been rational and at work for some weeks, when, without any apparent cause, except some disorder of the chylopoietic viscera, which it is probable existed, though un-known, she became excited, talked to herself, and was constantly moving about. Considerable increase of heat was found in the head, but the pulse exhibited no variation; it was only seventy, and of natural strength. She has had sleepless nights. An emetic and aperient were given; the head was shaved, and cold lotion applied; which much relieved her in a few days.

F. G. has been subject to paroxysms of mania for several years. Having recovered from one, and been sufficiently well to go to work for some weeks, the excitement again came on. His head was found hot, but the pulse only sixty. Aperients, and the cold application to the shaved head, soon removed it.

I could insert a catalogue of cases, in addition to those just mentioned, to show that although the commencement of insanity and any exacerbation of it in the old cases are attended almost invariably (indeed I think I should be justified in saying universally) with increased heat in the head : yet the alteration in the pulse is by no means without exception. In fact, I am fully convinced that from the rapidity of the pulse alone we can derive no information whatever. In many cases it seems to depend entirely upon causes purely nervous. I have known it vary in the same patient, during a single visit, as much as forty strokes, and be reduced from one hundred and twenty to eighty.

This heat in ordinary cases extends over the entire surface of the cranium, though in many instances particular portions of it are of a higher temperature than the other parts.*

The heat in the head is very generally accompanied by cold extremities. Want of sleep has been already mentioned. A cold clammy perspiration, accompanied with a peculiar fœtor, often referred to by writers on this subject, is certainly found in many patients. It gives the skin an appearance of having been rubbed over by some greasy substance : it varies very much in the same patient; and is most perceptible when the individual is labouring under a severe paroxysm. It is, however, by no means an universal accompaniment of mental derangement. A great number of patients, both of those who have recovered and those who have died, have never

---

* On this subject the medical reader is referred to the Notes.

exhibited it; but where it is found it invariably denotes the existence of organic disease in the brain; I do not recollect a single instance of a patient with this symptom having recovered : and on dissection, the ventricles have uniformly been filled with a great excess of water. The unpleasantness of this fœtor may be very much obviated by the constant use of the tepid bath.

A great want of nervous sensibility is another very frequent symptom. To such a degree will this exist, that diseases of the most painful nature, such as inflammation in the abdomen, in which all the viscera have, to a certain degree, been affected, have, upon *post mortem* inspections, been most unexpectedly discovered in those patients who neither complained nor appeared to suffer during their lives from this cause.

This want of sensibility enables them to endure that, without shrinking, which in the ordinary state of the nervous system would be attended with the most acute pain.

If those cases of insanity which have come on suddenly, with much cerebral disturbance, be left to themselves, or active measures be not immediately applied, before death takes place the result very frequently is such a state of diseased organization that some of the nerves of the senses, as well as those parts of the brain necessary for the mental manifestations, lose their specific action. Heat and cold cease to produce their usual effects ; the nerves of taste are so far injured, that the patient will eat his own ordure and drink his own urine, without even apparently discovering any thing offensive.

The opposite to this want of sensibility in the nerves of the five senses, is, however, not unfrequently a symptom of insanity. Both the optic and auditory nerves, as well as those of sensation, are frequently seen to be painfully acute, and give rise to many expressions of extravagant feeling, which, I believe, are really experienced by the patient, but which cannot be understood by those to whom they are related.

In many cases of insanity extreme hunger is observed to form a very striking feature. This arises from the great mental exertion which is kept up, often for days and weeks together, and when it is accompanied by much talking, as is frequently the case, great thirst is endured as well as hunger. But occasionally the reverse of this takes place, and the patient appears neither to require food nor drink, and sometimes obstinately refuses both for days together. This I suppose to arise from the secretions being altogether faulty, for the bowels, kidneys, &c. seem to be at such times almost in a total state of inaction.

It will be observed that many of the various symptoms previously enumerated are mentioned as accompanying insanity without any reference to the particular cause of the disease. In fact, whatever may have been the cause, the immediate effect is an excess

of blood in some portion, or in the whole of the brain
and its membranes, except in the cases where it
has been the result of loss of blood or excessive
bodily weakness. These cases are of rare occurrence, and easily distinguishable from those, the
general symptoms of which we have been describing.*

* The medical reader is referred to the Notes.

CHAPTER V.

ON IDIOCY AND FATUITY.

In treating on this subject, we shall confine the use of the term Idiocy to those cases, where the deficiency of understanding is congenital.

I make this distinction, because many patients during attacks of insanity exhibit appearances so closely resembling idiocy, that they are often considered incurable, and allowed to sink without an effort being made for their recovery. But no case, however apparently desperate, unless connate, will justify the neglect of the most strenuous exertions. Several cases under my care have recovered, where the patients have, on their admission, exhibited a total deprivation of all the mental faculties; and have been sent to the asylum only because their habits have become so dirty and offensive as to be a nuisance to the workhouses, where they had been previously confined.

The following is a striking instance in which, from the fatuous appearance of the patient, he might have been considered so decidedly incurable as to be left without any effort being made or thought possible to be of use : but he ultimately got well.

J. P., about twenty-four years of age, had been insane about twelve months when admitted. He had had an attack some time before, but the particular circumstances connected with it are not known. At the time of his admission he appeared fast sinking into fatuity. He was silent and melancholy, sitting for the whole day in one place and position unless roused; apparently unconscious of all surrounding objects, and scarcely any thing could induce him either to move or speak. In this state he continued for some months, notwithstanding every effort was made to engage him in some employment. By perseverance, however, he was at last induced to assist a little in cleaning the ward : no sooner had he began this trifling occupation than an improvement took place in his mental faculties ; his countenance assumed a more cheerful aspect, his spirits were more lively, and manners obliging. At the end of seven months, from his beginning to work, he was discharged cured, much to the delight of his relatives, and the astonishment of every one who saw him at his first admission.

T. T., about fifty years of age, was found wandering in the street, and sent to the house of correction as a vagrant. He was perfectly unconscious of every thing around him, and appeared idiotic. In this state he was sent to the asylum.

Though grey-headed, and looking much older than he really was, he had still the remains of a fine person; he was upwards of six feet high, with a countenance and form of head presenting a striking contrast with his imbecile state of mind. He was in good bodily health, and free from all appearance of disease, except a small ulcer on the leg. He was placed amongst the idiotic patients, and was apparently sinking into the last state of fatuity. All the information that could be obtained respecting him was that he had been a soldier. I attempted day after day to induce him to enter into conversation, but in vain. "I have been a soldier," was the most he would say. Many weeks elapsed without any improvement taking place, and his case was considered quite hopeless. A change for the better took place very suddenly. Without any previous conversation with any one, he requested the keeper to give him a sheet of paper, on which he wrote the following letter :—

"MADAM,

"I feel myself completely at a loss for an apology, which would in any way justify the liberty I am now taking. Not personally known to you, I feel the great awkwardness of addressing you, particularly in the character of a petitioner.

"I know not indeed whether I can do better than state the circumstances which have induced me to adopt this measure.

"Some time ago, driven by the greatest distress, I addressed myself to your husband, hoping that in consideration of our former intimacy he would have afforded me some assistance. I remained a fortnight in London without receiving any answer—indeed I have no means of knowing whether this letter reached him. Since that time I have been a miserable wretched wanderer through the country, without friends and without shelter. Such were the severity of my sufferings that my intellects became unhinged, and I am indebted to the charity of this establishment for the continuance of my wretched existence, and the prospect of being once again enabled to mix in society. Whether either the one or the other will be beneficial I have my doubts. When discharged from this house I have no prospect but of again becoming a wretched wanderer, without resources, and destitute of friends. The prospect is truly deplorable, and yet such, in a very short time, must be my fate.

"These, madam, are the melancholy circumstances which have induced me to endeavour to interest you in my fate, a measure I never should have adopted if I had not been fearful of a letter to your husband sharing the same fate as my last.

"I will not intrude further on your time than merely intreating you to pardon me for the liberty I have taken, assuring yourself that nothing but the most extreme distress and despair could have driven me to it. Should your humanity be so far interested as to induce you to afford me any assistance, believe me it will be most thankfully and gratefully received."

Not receiving any answer to the above, the following was sent to a gentleman who very kindly assisted him.

"MY DEAR SIR,

"I know not how again to intrude on you with a tale of disaster and woe, yet your kind expressions, and still kinder manner, when I quitted you, are so strongly imprinted on my recollection, that I cannot help flattering myself you will not be offended with my present application to you. Yet it seems unfair, that, because you have once befriended me, I should again harass you with my misfortunes, again solicit a renewal of kindness, to which I feel perfectly conscious I have no claim, except what the benevolence of your heart allows to those unfortunate beings whom you may once have known in better circumstances.

"The vivid remembrance of the peculiarly heartfelt tenderness of your manner to me, when at ——, emboldens me to do what it is impossible to apologize for, unless you will admit, as an excuse, the truly pitiable situation in which I am at present placed. When I left —— I made several attempts in ——, and afterwards in London and its neighbourhood, to obtain some employment which would

afford me the means of supporting an existence
which was daily becoming more and more burthen-
some. I will not harass your feelings by the
melancholy detail of the miseries I endured during
this fruitless search ; suffice it to say, that after
several days of misery the most exquisite, without
shelter and without food, I was taken out of the
Serpentine River, and conveyed to —— workhouse.
There I was discovered by a gentleman, an old
schoolfellow, who kindly supplied me with some
clothes and a little money, with which, by his advice,
I set out for the north of England, with the hope
that there, amongst those I had formerly known, I
might obtain some situation that would afford me
the necessaries of life. At —— in —— I was
taken ill, and so long confined that my small stock
of money was nearly exhausted ; when somewhat
recovered, though in a very weak state, I again bent
my course northward, and have some recollection of
having been in Newark, Retford, and Doncaster,
but for many succeeding months my existence is a
perfect blank, as far as my own recollection is concerned. I have since learnt that about —— I was
found wandering in the streets of ——, a perfect
lunatic, and by the magistrates sent to ——, where
I have been taken care of ever since with the
greatest possible kindness ; and am now declared, by
the physicians, to be perfectly sane. Indeed I feel
conscious that my mental faculties are completely
restored, for I am again capable of contemplating

and feeling, with the most acute sensibility, my truly forlorn and friendless situation. Something, however, must be done; and it is my intention to go down into the north and endeavour to obtain some employment, however humble, that will keep me from starving : but I am almost destitute of clothing and money! Can you? will you, dear ——, assist me ? I feel the blush of shame burning on my cheek whilst I make the request, but the most urgent, the most miserable necessity impels me. Forgive and pardon your forlorn, unhappy friend."

These letters are inserted to show how much talent may yet exist when every faculty appears dead, and as a stimulus to relax no effort to kindle into a blaze the sparks of mind that may yet remain. In this instance, under the semblance of hopeless fatuity, was hid mental power of the highest order.

It is scarcely necessary to say, that an inquiry was immediately made into every particular concerning him : when it turned out that he had received a liberal education, that he had been brought up in expectation of having a very large fortune, but his relative on whom he depended had died poor. He had a sufficiency to procure him a commission in the army, and had been in India. He was an elegant scholar, with fascinating manners, but unhappily was devoid of those high religious principles without which the most brilliant talents tend but to the destruction both of the possessors and of others.

He left the asylum quite well, and procured a situation which he retained for some years.

Idiocy arises, either from the brain being defective in size and power, where all the mental manifestations are found imperfect, and the functions of automatic life alone seem to be performed; or from a brain of a natural size having some organic disease or mal-conformation. In these cases, some of the faculties are often particularly active, but so unduly balanced as to render the individual unfit to be at large.

Idiots are very frequently subject to epilepsy, and many of them are highly mischievous, furious, and obscene. As far as I have had an opportunity of observing, they are not long-lived.

In such cases, it is needless to say, no medical remedies exist. But much may be done by proper care and moral treatment, to check the evil propensities, and to bring forward the good in proportion to the powers : these vary from the mere capability of swallowing food to that of behaving with propriety in the ordinary scenes of life.

Fatuity, which is the result of insanity, is, in its symptoms and consequences, the same as idiocy, the only difference being that in the idiotic the faculties were from birth imperfect, and that in the fatuous there was a period when the functions were performed in a healthy manner. This fatuity sometimes arises from long-continued over-excited cerebral action. Another not infrequent cause is the weakness arising from excessive general bleedings and evacuations in cases of mania. The medical reader is referred to the notes for an account of by far the most usual cause.

CHAPTER VI.

ON THE TREATMENT OF INSANITY.

WE have now come to the most important part of our subject, the previous chapters being only introductory, and intended to throw such a light upon insanity as to enable us to ward off an attack, or to proceed in the treatment of it on rational principles. It is of course impossible to lay down any particular plan to be adopted in all cases. In those instances where the causes of the disease and the circumstances of the patient are the most similar, constitutional differences exist, which make variations in the treatment absolutely necessary, and which require the most watchful care and discrimination on the part of the physician. It will be the object of this chapter to make a classification of those cases in which the same system, modified according to individual circumstances, ought to be adopted; and to point out the general principles of treatment applicable to each class.

As insanity has been considered, in all cases, to be a disease of the brain or nervous system, one of

the most obvious divisions will be according to the
nature of the disease which exists there.   We shall
therefore divide the subject into two classes; one,
where diseased action only is going on in the brain,
and the other, where the continuance of the diseased
action has produced diseased organization.   The
first class I shall call incipient, and the latter
chronic insanity.   It ought not to be forgotten that
cure, or much relief, is to be expected only whilst
the disease is incipient.   If lesion of the brain once
takes place, however the consequence of it may be
palliated, and the patient rendered moderately comfortable, the mental manifestations can never be
completely restored.   There is a great objection
to the usual division of insanity into mania and
melancholia : it is apt to mislead.   These are but
symptoms and results of over-exercise of different
mental faculties ; and they are alike attended with
excess of sanguineous circulation in the brain.   It
may be of material assistance to our forming correct
views of the treatment to be adopted, shortly to
analyze and trace the probable steps of the disease.
Now, except in the cases of insanity arising from
loss of blood, want of nutrition, or some other
debilitating cause, in a very large proportion of post-
mortem examinations of persons who have died
insane, whatever may have been the cause of the
disease, the appearance of the brain clearly indicates
the previous existence there for a considerable
period of inflammatory action, that is, of an excess of

blood. May we not then infer, that, with the exception of the cases alluded to, insanity, whatever may be its primary cause, begins with an excess of sanguiferous circulation in the brain, or in some part of it; and that, from the continuance of this accelerated circulation, a morbid change of structure takes place, not only in the part of the brain at first attacked, but gradually and eventually in the whole mass of the brain and its membranes; and that the effusion of serum under the membranes and in the ventricles, almost universally found in old cases, is the ultimate result of this excessive sanguineous circulation. The mere fact, that in cases where the disease has been coming on gradually and almost imperceptibly for many months or years, no appearance of inflammatory action has been observed during its progress, is no evidence that a measure of excessive sanguiferous action, proportionate to the gradual change in the conduct and sentiments, has not existed. The immediate cause of this excess of circulation is either over-exercise of the brain or of some part of it, or irritation produced in it by its sympathy with some other diseased bodily organ. In the former case, an undue quantity of blood is required and supplied; and in the latter, the results are the same as in any other cases of irritation.

It may be objected to this theory, that patients frequently do not complain of pain in any part of the head. Now, in nine cases out of ten, on the *com-*

mencement of the disease, they do complain of heaviness and pain there.   This is the fact, with scarcely an exception, when the disease comes on suddenly ; but after the diseased action has continued for some time the parts seem to accommodate themselves to the change, and this pain is no longer felt.   Indeed, as has been previously observed, diseased organization may exist to a very great extent without being accompanied by any pain.   Supposing then this to be the mode in which the brain is affected, it obviously becomes of the greatest importance to ascertain, if possible, what is the cause which immediately produces this increased circulation. Although bleeding and other medical treatment may for a time prevent an excessive volume of blood from being sent through the brain, yet if the cause remains, and a part of the brain continues to be excited to undue exercise, or to be irritated by sympathy, it will demand and receive more than its due and healthy share of blood from the system. Mischievous and fatal results constantly arise in practice from want of attention to the cause of this increased circulation, particularly in cases of mania. Very copious evacuations and profuse bleedings from the system are resorted to, and after the animal strength of the patient is exhausted, he becomes quiet, but the mental delusion still remains.   Supposing the cause of the disease to be a permanent one, such as any moral cause, the brain, or a portion of it, continues to be unduly exercised, and to obtain from the system more than its due share of the blood, which the lancet has left. But when the loss of blood has been excessive, the vital power, in numerous instances, is never recovered, and the patient either dies or sinks into a state of fatuity. Unfortunately many of the patients received into public hospitals, as recent cases, have previously undergone this exhausting process. The constitution has not energy to rally, and there is, in consequence of this injudicious treatment, a much greater mortality amongst the recent cases than amongst the old, in proportion to their numbers and ages. In fact, if the cause be permanent, there is a greater probability of ultimate cure, when nature is left to herself, and the violence of the attack allowed to be expended, without any attempt at relief, than where her powers have been wasted by *excessive* depletions. On the first appearance therefore of any of the symptoms mentioned in the foregoing chapter, the attention ought to be most carefully directed to the ascertaining, if possible, and then removing the cause. Although the diseased action may not immediately cease on its removal, yet there can be but little hope of cure whilst it continues to operate. It has been already shown, that the brain and nervous system may be affected either primarily or by sympathy. Amongst the primary causes of disease, blows and other direct physical injuries have been enumerated; but the brain, unlike any other organ of the body, is idiophatically liable to diseased action from moral, as well as from physical causes: whilst diseased action in the stomach, liver, uterus, &c., when induced by moral causes, is only the result of sympathy with the disordered brain or nervous system. But although similar symptoms of inflammation and irritation will be observed, whatever may have been the cause, it is obvious that diseased action in the brain, arising from blows, fevers, tumours, or from the pressure of spiculi of bone, will require a treatment different from that which ought to be adopted where it is the result of over-action brought on by jealousy, too great anxiety on religious subjects, or any other constantly operating moral cause. In the former class of cases, moral remedies would be useless, and physical ones must be applied ; in the latter, medical treatment is only useful to allay irritation, and to counteract the physical injury produced by the action of the moral cause. The grand object to be attained, with a view to ultimate cure, is the removing the cause by moral treatment. Again, cases of insanity arising from diseased action of the brain, produced by its sympathy with some other diseased bodily organ, clearly require a peculiar mode of treatment. Some of the physical causes of insanity may be only of short duration, and may cease almost immediately after the diseased action in the brain has been produced ; whilst the moral causes of insanity, with scarcely any exception, and other of the physical causes, may be permanent, and may continue to exert their baneful influence long after the commencement of the attack. The first step is to ascertain the cause, and this can only be done by careful inquiries of the friends of the patient. There is usually not much difficulty in the investigation, when insanity has been the result of a blow on the head, or of any other direct physical injury, or where it has been the consequence of any very marked and notorious change of circumstances : but when the alteration in the conduct, or mental manifestations, has been very gradual, and no hereditary tendency to the disease has existed, and there have not been any peculiar circumstances likely to produce an over-exertion of the brain, or of any part of it, the inquiry becomes more difficult. In the latter cases, sympathy with some of the disordered viscera will very probably be found to be the cause of the disease.

One circumstance frequently exists in the beginning of this disease, which may account for many of the mistakes usually fallen into in its early treatment : and that is, the perfect state of action in which the greater part, if not all but one or two, of the organs remain. So that unless these are frequently wanted for the performance of the ordinary duties of life, diseased action may go on for a long time without being discovered. To use a figure, I would compare the brain to a piano-forte ; and the feelings, passions, and various faculties, to the different strings. One or two of the notes may be out of tune from over work, or it may happen from being formed of a more delicate material than the rest; but as the note which is out of tune does not prevent the others from giving their correct sound, the instrument may be continued in use for a long time, without its being thought absolutely necessary to have it repaired : although when the defect is observed, no one would expect that it would ever regain its proper tone again until properly mended. Something similar to this takes place in a very large proportion of cases of insanity, with this difference, that the piano has no power whatever within itself to repair the mischief. Happily for man, not only in this, but in most other diseases, the constitution possesses a vis medicatrix, which works by itself, and often accomplishes its purpose in spite of our ignorance and blunders. Many indeed are the cases of insanity cured in this way. The diseased action spends itself, the brain recovers its tone, and the functions are performed as before : although in other instances there is not sufficient constitutional vigour to restore the healthy action, and the disease, being neglected, gradually extends to other portions of the brain. This is very constantly the case where the insanity has first shown itself in some slight and gradual alteration in the conduct or moral manifestations. As the patients are tolerably manageable, no steps are taken to cure the disease, and many months constantly elapse before they are placed under proper medical care. Now, reasoning from analogy on the effects of disease of any other organ continued for so long a period, it must be expected that the disease will be difficult of cure, and that, when the brain is restored to its healthy action, it will still be weak, and will retain a liability to be again attacked in the same way; especially if the same exciting cause is applied which first brought on the disease, or, indeed, if from any other reason it be over-worked. It is well known that some persons are liable, whenever ill, to have peculiar parts affected; and that many have periodical attacks of the same disease, especially if they have once laboured under any severe and long attack. This is precisely the case with regard to insanity. It is liable to recur; it frequently comes on periodically; and in this, as well as in other diseases, as the organ becomes gradually weakened, so it requires less and less to create disturbance in its action. It sometimes happens, that, on the very first attack, some part has suffered so much as never perfectly to regain its functions; and if this is one, upon the right action of which the moral conduct is much influenced, the patient must necessarily be subject to such a degree of restraint as is necessary for his own well-being and that of others : but certainly to no more. It most frequently however happens, that the diseased action is so subdued, that the faculties resume their former power, and continue in healthy action, either altogether, which is unfor-

tunately not often the case, where the disease has
been suffered for a considerable time to remain
neglected, or for longer or shorter periods, as the
excitability of the parts is greater or less.

Supposing the cause to be ascertained, let us next
consider the treatment of Incipient Insanity. We
shall first direct our attention to cases, where the
disease is attended with an excess of sanguiferous
circulation in the brain, classifying these, according
to their causes, into cases, where it is produced by a
direct physical injury, or by some sudden increase
of general sanguiferous circulation, arising from a
merely temporary cause ; secondly, into the cases
where the brain is primarily affected by the action
of some moral cause ; and, thirdly, into the cases
where the insanity is caused by the brain sympathizing with some other disordered organ.

Having considered incipient insanity, attended
with excess of sanguiferous circulation, the treatment of it, when it is the result of a want of an
adequate supply of blood to the brain, will next
follow ; and under this head will be included the
cases of insanity arising from the vice previously
referred to ; as whatever may be the increase of
circulation in the cerebellum, the cerebrum does
not in these cases appear to receive its due share.
Indeed, as they require a peculiar treatment distinct from that where the disease arises from any
other cause, the arrangement is unimportant ; and
they seem to fall more naturally into this division of

the subject than in those previously mentioned.
The mode of treatment, when the disease is chronic,
will lastly fall under our notice. Let us commence
with cases of insanity arising from blows on the
head, *coup-de-soleil*, &c. It frequently happens,
that injuries inflicted upon the head produce at
the time comparatively little disturbance in the
constitution; and consequently little immediate
attention is paid to them. These, it is well known,
are often followed by acute inflammation some
days after the accident, and subsequently by death.
Sometimes, instead of phrenitis coming on, the
first symptom of any real injury having been sustained is shown in some altered manner in the
conduct or sentiments of the patient. At the same
time, that there are often wildness of expression,
irritability of manner, foul tongue, costive bowels,
a quickened pulse, and sleepless nights. If, in this
early stage of the disease, these symptoms be considered to arise from the accident, and medical advice
be resorted to, subsequent insanity may be prevented as easily as high inflammatory action of any
other organ. At the commencement of an attack
of this kind, depletion may be used, according to the
strength of the patient, very freely; and much more
so than in cases of insanity arising from moral
causes. Copious bleeding from the temporal artery,
free purging with calomel and extract of colocynth,
and cold applications to the shaved head, are the
means most to be depended upon; the patient taking,

at the same time, nitrate of potash in ten-grain
doses, with small nauseating doses of tartar emetic :
the extremities being kept warm with bottles of hot
water, or even stimulated with mustard poultices.
The apartments should be kept well ventilated, but
all noise and light should be carefully excluded.
After such a quantity of blood has been drawn from
the system as the constitution is thought capable of
bearing, if the inflammatory action still continues
violent, local bleeding may follow, either by leeches
or cupping as may be convenient, and digitalis
given in conjunction with the nitrate of potash.
But in the use of digitalis great caution ought to
be observed as to the dose.   I have heard of a
drachm of the tincture being given at once, and even
repeated in that quantity.   I can only say, that I
have seen very serious consequences arise from much
smaller doses ; and I generally find that, independently of avoiding the dangerous results of large
doses, smaller ones, more frequently repeated, produce a more lasting and salutary effect.   Indeed not
only in insanity, but in all diseases in which the
nervous system is much implicated, the operation of
digitalis is so uncertain, that the greatest watchfulness should be used whilst it is administered.   From
five to ten drops, repeated three or four times a day,
is as much as we ever begin with.   The dose may
be increased as the necessity of the case and the
strength of the patient justify : but it should ever
be remembered, that the debilitating effects arising

even from small doses, if they have been taken for some time, take place very suddenly; and the most extraordinary prostration of strength often follows. From this prostration of strength no stimulus seems sufficient to recover the patient. If the above remedies are commenced in the early stage, and carefully followed up, as the strength of the patient will bear them, the recovery may take place rapidly; and there will be no occasion to remove such patient from home, and the immediate care and attention of his relations and friends. It not unfrequently happens that the stomach becomes so weakened by the use of the means requisite to reduce inflammatory action, that it cannot digest the food required to restore the system to its usual strength. Bitters, stimulating tonics, and exercise in the open air, are necessary in this stage of the disease. Where the patient, notwithstanding the application of the remedies above mentioned, does not recover, the symptoms and treatment become so nearly similar to those where the insanity arises from moral causes, that it will be unnecessary to detail them here. If any portion of the bone is depressed, the pressure must of course be removed before any other remedy is attempted. A curious instance of the importance of attending to this is mentioned by Sir A. Cooper. " A man was pressed on board one of his Majesty's ships, early in the late revolutionary war. While on board this vessel, in the Mediterranean, he received a fall from the yard-arm, and when he was picked up he was found to be insensible. The vessel soon after making Gibraltar, he was deposited in an hospital in that place, where he remained for some months, still insensible; and some time after he was brought from Gibraltar, on board the *Dolphin* frigate, to a depôt for sailors at Deptford. While he was at Deptford, the surgeon under whose care he was, was visited by Mr. Davy. The surgeon said to Mr. Davy, ' I have a case which I think you would like to see; it is a man who has been insensible for many months; he lies on his back, with very few signs of life; he breathes, indeed, has a pulse, and some motion in his fingers; but in all other respects he is apparently deprived of all powers of mind, volition or sensation.' Mr. Davy, on examining the patient, found that there was a slight depression on one part of the head. Being informed of the accident, which had occasioned this depression, he recommended the man to be sent to St. Thomas's Hospital. He was placed under the care of Mr. Cline, and when he was first admitted into this hospital I saw him lying on his back, breathing without any great difficulty; his pulse regular, his arms extended, and his fingers moving to and fro to the motion of his heart; so that you could count his pulse by this motion of his fingers. If he wanted food, he had the power of moving his lips and tongue; and this action of his mouth was the signal to his attendants for supplying this want.

" Mr. Cline, on examining his head, found an obvious depression ; and thirteen months and a few days after the accident he was carried into the operating theatre, and there trepanned. The depressed portion of bone was elevated from the skull. While he was lying on the table the motion of his fingers went on, during the operation, but no sooner was the portion of the bone raised than it ceased. The operation was performed at one o'clock in the afternoon ; and, at four o'clock, as I was walking through the wards, I went up to the man's bedside, and was surprised to see him sitting up in his bed. He had raised himself on his pillow : I asked him if he felt any pain, and he immediately put his hand to his head. This showed that volition and sensation were returning. In four days from that time the man was able to get out of bed, and began to converse ; and in a few days more he was able to tell us where he came from.

" He recollected the circumstance of his having been pressed, and carried down to Plymouth or Falmouth ; but from that moment, up to the time when the operation was performed, that is, for a period of thirteen months and some days, his mind had remained in a state of perfect oblivion :—he had drunk, as it were, the cup of Lethe ; he had suffered a complete death as far as regarded his mental, and almost all his bodily powers ; but, by removing a small portion of bone with the saw, he was at once restored to all the functions of his mind, and almost all the powers of his body."

Insanity, arising from coup-de-soleil, evidently proceeds from a physical cause acting immediately on the brain. Such cases are not very common in this country. Coup-de-soleil more frequently causes frenzy and death than insanity : diseased action of the brain is, however, very frequently brought on by long-continued exposure to heat and the rays of the sun ; but not in so sudden a manner as when it takes place immediately from coup-de-soleil. Whenever disease of the brain does occur from this cause, no time should be lost in the vigorous application of the foregoing remedies. We have reason to believe that diseased action in the brain, arising from this cause, proceeds much more rapidly than from most others. As far as my experience extends, I have not seen any advantage arise from the use of blisters upon the head, especially during the paroxysm ; they appear rather to create irritation than to allay it ; and they prevent, by their application, the use of ice or cold water, which has often the most salutary and instantaneous effect. It has not unfrequently occurred to us, that when the diseased action has existed to such an excess, as to have prevented the patient sleeping for several days and nights, upon the head being shaved and cold applied to it, at the same time that warmth has been used to the extremities, he has almost instantaneously fallen asleep. If the disease continues, a mode of treatment similar to that which will be hereafter prescribed for cases, where the insanity has arisen from moral causes, must be adopted.

The only cases of insanity arising from excess of general sanguiferous circulation, from a merely temporary cause, are, in the instances where it is produced by a continuance, for several days, of a state of intoxication. When the patient is strong, and the system not previously debilitated by a habit of spirit-drinking, a treatment similar to the one just pointed out may be successfully adopted. Sudden depletion, and to a very considerable extent, may have a salutary effect.

I recollect a case which occurred to me thirty-five years ago, of a seaman, who had been living in a very intemperate way for some time, until he became so maniacal that he could not be kept on board his ship. He was sent to the workhouse at Hull, where he had only been a few days when he leaped out of the window; in consequence, as he afterwards related to me, of believing that the devil wanted to get possession of him. He thought he should escape him if he could but get out of the house. He said he felt quite free for some time, but he at last heard him beneath the pavement, wherever he went in the town. He then thought, that, if he could only leap on board a ship, which was at some little distance from the wharf, he should avoid him; but he had not been long on

board before he felt convinced that he was scratch-
ing at the bottom of the vessel, and it then occurred to him, that if he got on shore and cut his
throat, he should be safe.   He borrowed a knife
from a sailor, whom he met, and instantly cut
his throat from ear to ear.   As is very usual in
these attempts at self-destruction, the pharynx was
wounded, but the carotids were uninjured; the
hemorrhage from the superficial vessels was enormous.   The parts were speedily brought together;
the wound healed by the first intention : he was
never insane one moment after the brain was relieved by the immediate loss of blood.   He related
to me all the above circumstances;—he got perfectly well, and went to sea, within a month after
his unsuccessful attempt at self-destruction.   In
this case we have seen the sudden good effects of a
very large and copious bleeding, as in other inflammatory diseases requiring such treatment; and, as
no exciting cause continued to act upon the organ,
after the first unintended remedy had been applied,
the man got well.

As most of the cases arising from this class of
causes are attended with mania, and considerable
violence, it may not be out of place to observe, that
in all cases where the patient begins to be ungo-
vernable, the kindest and least afflicting mode of
proceeding, even to the patient himself, is to procure such an overwhelming power to restrain him,
as to make him feel it useless to resist.   Very few

indeed will contend with three or four determined
persons; but if only one or two be present, the most
violent opposition is made. The most simple and
least objectionable mode of confinement, is that of a
pair of wide canvass sleeves, connected by a broad
canvass shoulder-strap, so as to rest easily on the
shoulders. They ought to come up well on the
shoulders, and to extend about an inch beyond the
ends of the fingers: the part covering the hand
should be made of tolerably stiff leather, to prevent
the hand grasping any thing. They keep the arms
hanging easily, and in a natural position, by the
sides of the body. They are fastened at the back
by two straps, one going from one sleeve a little
above the elbow, across the loins to a similar position in the other sleeve; a second lower down, and
by three similar straps in the front; the latter being
secured by buckles, which, in large establishments,
where there are many patients to be attended to
by one keeper, ought to be locked. This mode of
fastening has many advantages over the straight-
waistcoat. In the first place, it is less heating, it
produces no pressure upon the chest, and the arms,
though secured from mischief, have so much freedom that the blood can circulate freely; as with
these sleeves ligatures of every description are
unnecessary. It is sometimes also requisite to
secure the feet. For this purpose we find, that a
couple of leathern straps well lined with wool,
placed round the ankles, and secured to the bed by

staples, is all that is necessary. In hospital practice cases will sometimes occur, where it may be necessary to secure the bedding in its place. This can be done by having a thick quilt fastened over the blankets, by three leathern straps, to the sides of the bed. It occasionally happens, that, unless this precaution is taken, the patient will toss all the clothes off from the bed. In the winter season such a circumstance may be attended with bad consequences, if the patient is not very frequently seen. It cannot be too deeply impressed upon the minds of all who have any management of the insane, that in the application of these, or any other coercive measures, the greatest mildness and forbearance should be used towards the unhappy sufferers. Though it may be necessary, in some cases, to assemble such a force that the appearance of the persons alone may prevent all opposition, yet it is unwise and cruel for the whole party to fly at the poor patient, to accomplish that which may be frequently done under the soothing influence of one favoured attendant; the mind of the patient being subdued by the presence of the others, who are ready to render further assistance if required.

Another very convenient and easy mode of confinement, is, by an arm-chair. Each of the arms of the chair forms a padded box, which incloses the arm of the patient, from a little below the elbow to the wrist. The box ought to be sufficiently large to contain the arm quite loosely, and without any pressure, and the hand will remain at liberty. A board, which forms a very convenient rest, is attached by hinges to the inner side of one of the arms of the chair, and is fastened to the other arm. When the confinement of the arms is unnecessary the box may be opened, and the patient may still remain fastened in the chair, by means of a loose strap passing in the front of the body, through two holes at the back of the chair, and there buckled. The chair may be fitted with a foot-board, a little elevated above the floor, and perforated with holes. Under this board a vessel constantly filled with hot water, ought to be kept, in cold weather.

The cases of insanity, which arise from any physical cause, not producing organic disease in the brain or nervous system, vary in their duration from one to six months, in proportion as the disease is attended to or neglected, on its first appearance.

We will next consider the treatment of cases of insanity arising from moral causes. In these cases the diseased action in the brain is rarely produced by any sudden shock, but it generally arises from the continued operation of some exciting cause, producing excessive vascular action in the brain, or in some part of it. Unfortunately, the alteration in the sentiments and conduct, in many cases, is so gradual, that diseased action in the brain may have existed without being suspected, until diseased organization has actually taken place. When the insanity is discovered, it is rarely in the power of the physician immediately to remove the cause. It is however necessary, from time to time, to apply such physical remedies as may relieve the system, and prevent the diseased action from terminating in diseased organization; and, at the same time, to adopt every moral means of placing the patient out of the immediate influence of the primary cause of the disease. The treatment, therefore, of this class of cases, will necessarily be divided into medical and moral. Let us consider these divisions separately. First, then, as to the medical treatment. In *all* cases of insanity arising from moral causes, on the *commencement* of the diseased action of the brain, more or less disorder will be found to exist in some of the other bodily functions. After the diseased action in the brain has continued for some time and become chronic, the other functions, in many cases, gradually recover their tone; and when lesion of the brain has taken place, the patients frequently enjoy a fair state of health. But until the system has become habituated to the diseased action of the brain, some other part of the body, varying, according to the different idiosyncrasies of the individual, will be affected by sympathy. The functions of the stomach, liver, bowels, or kidneys are usually disordered; and it becomes necessary to adopt the proper medical means to restore them to right action. These means, with the exception which will be shortly noticed, are such as are usually employed when the same diseases have come on from any other cause. At the same time, the excess of sanguineous circulation in the brain, which is the immediate cause of their derangement, should be diminished. We will point out the medical remedies to effect the latter object. In the treatment of insanity, arising from physical injuries, it has been seen, that very large bleedings and copious evacuations are frequently of great use : but this is not the case in insanity from moral causes. In these cases, although there exists an excess of blood in the brain, yet, as this arises from the brain, or some part of it being constantly over excited, and therefore receiving more than its due share of blood from the system, the withdrawing any portion from the system generally will not alter the proportion which the brain will appropriate to itself, during the continuance of the exciting cause. But, in consequence of this extra exertion of the brain, the constitution needs all its vital energy for its support. In the treatment, then, of insanity arising from moral causes, no greater quantity of blood ought to be abstracted, than that which will be sufficient so to reduce the inflammatory action in the brain, as from time to time to relieve the vessels, and prevent the coming on of diseased organization ; and, of course, the more directly the blood is taken from the diseased part, the less it will be requisite to abstract. In fact, the constitution and system generally require supporting, in consequence of the excessive exertion ; whilst the part of the brain locally affected with inflammatory action, requires that the gorged vessels should be relieved of their load to prevent lesion.   As the first means, then, of diminishing the circulation, the head should be shaved, and the parts of the scalp, under which it is probable the excess of circulation is taking place, should be repeatedly bled with leeches, or cupped, a small quantity of blood only being abstracted at each time of bleeding.   In many cases, the parts of the scalp to which the leeches or cupping-glasses may be applied, so as to produce the greatest local benefit, with the least expense to the constitution, may be discovered by the presence of additional heat or pain; but in some instances the temperature of the scalp is equable, and the patient refuses to give any information as to his feelings.   In these cases, the only means of ascertaining the part of the brain which is disordered, is by noting the mode in which the altered conduct or sentiment exhibits itself. In many cases, where the insanity has been clearly confined to particular propensities, I have found a greater degree of heat in the scalp covering that region of the brain which phrenologists have assigned as the organs of such propensities, than in other parts of the scalp, and the patient has complained of such parts being the seat of pain.   I say region, because I wish it to be particularly noticed, that I do not pretend that, in any case, the heat is quite circumscribed to the particular convolution of the brain affected.   Every one knows, that when inflammation takes place in any part of the body,

it is not confined entirely to the spot which is diseased. Gout may be fixed in the joint of the great
toe, but the parts of the foot immediately around it
will partake of the heat. In other cases, therefore,
where the patient is silent, if I find from the conduct, that a certain set of feelings and propensities
is deranged, I apply leeches or cupping-glasses to
the region pointed out by phrenologists as their
organs. I am convinced, from experience, that this
mode of applying leeches has been very generally
successful. I do not say, that if they had been
applied to other parts of the head, similar results
might not have followed ; but, in the absence of any
other means of finding out the particular seat of the
disease, when no variation in temperature exists,
and no particular pain is described, I have adopted
this method, and with success as to the ultimate
result.

In numerous chronic cases also, (the treatment of
which will be noticed hereafter,) where, from the
imperfect manner in which certain functions are
performed during the most healthy state of the
patient, there is every reason to believe that lesion
exists in some parts of the brain, an application of
leeches, or cupping-glasses, on a similar principle,
relieves the periodical exacerbations of the disease
to which they are liable, and very greatly shortens
their duration. But in these cases again, I am unable to say, that the application to other parts of the
head would not be attended with similar results :

as I should not think myself justified, for the purpose of any philosophical experiment, in neglecting the means which I really believe to be the best calculated to diminish the sufferings of the poorest or most imbecile patient under my care. Supposing, then, the head to have been shaved, and the leeches or glasses applied where, according to the judgment of the physician, they will most efficaciously relieve the vessels of the brain, the head ought to be kept cool by ice, or by cold applications. Ice is by far the best refrigerant. Every public institution for the cure of the insane ought to be provided with an ice-house. The ice is most conveniently applied by powdering it tolerably small, and then putting it into a cap made of water-proof cotton ; as that prevents it running down the neck and face when it dissolves. When no ice is to be obtained, cold water, or weak vinegar and water, may be substituted for it ; but cold applications of some kind on the shaven scalp ought to be most strenuously persevered in, until the head becomes cool. The shower-bath is frequently used in these cases, but I do not think with the same advantage as the continued cold applications. The re-action which takes place in some measure counterbalances the good which is derived from the temporary relief to the brain. The lower extremities ought to be kept warm ; and, if other means for that purpose be inefficient, mustard poultices may be applied with advantage to the feet, particularly in cases where the whole surface of the head is excessively hot. And there are cases in which the sanguineous circulation is so excessive, as to make it requisite to abstract blood from the system by the lancet, as well as from the scalp by leeches. As in other diseases, acute topical inflammation sometimes runs so high, as to make it requisite to abstract blood from a patient whose general health can ill bear depletion. Now it may be taken as a principle, that a person insane from moral causes is one who cannot, without injury to the constitution, bear depletion : and the lancet must be used with great caution even in the plethoric, and in those who are apparently the strongest. The local bleedings with leeches may be repeated as often as it is judged that the vessels require relief. Watchfulness forms so prominent a feature in almost all recent cases caused by direct action on the brain, that it is necessary to dwell rather more at large upon it. To allay irritation is evidently the great desideratum : but as it is well known that there are peculiar idiosyncrasies in almost every constitution, so it will be evident that the means must be varied as we find them to exist. The same medicine which will allay it in one will not in another; but, on the contrary, increase it. This is particularly the case with opium, which is rarely found admissible in insanity. It more frequently creates heat, and general febrile action, than procures sleep : if given at all, it should be in conjunction with ipecacuanha; from five to ten grains of which, taken at bed-time, is sometimes found useful—most probably from the action usually produced on the skin by this remedy. We find the application of cold to the shaved head to be the most effectual means, in the first stage of the disease, to procure sleep ; and, afterwards, useful exercise out of doors. I have repeatedly seen patients who had been in the most violent state of excitement, and entirely without sleep for many days and nights, notwithstanding every effort has been used to procure it by the administering various narcotics, and the use of hop pillows, sink into the most comfortable repose on using the pediluvium, and applying cold to the shaven head. I have sometimes thought, that the placing a patient on a bed, kept gently rocked by a person not in the room with him, might have a tendency to produce sleep. This might be easily contrived, but I have not tried its effect. In the first stage of the disease we ought, if possible, to avoid the use of narcotic medicines ; and to endeavour to procure sleep, by allaying irritation, in the method above pointed out. I wish particularly to press this, because much has been said by some authors, on the necessity of procuring sleep by any means ; and of keeping up the strength of the constitution with hearty suppers, porter and other stimulants. There is no doubt that a full meal very often produces sleep ; and, that in the more chronic stage of the disease the exhaustion is often very great, and the

constitution consequently requires an extra quantity
of food. If the patient, under these circumstances,
goes to bed with a stomach nearly empty, he will
get no sleep; but hearty suppers are not admissible
in the incipient stage. The diet should be low, if
the patient can bear it; but certainly, in this stage,
never stimulating. It may in general be confined
to gruel, milk, and pudding. Balm tea is the most
refreshing diluent the patient can take to allay the
thirst, which is usually suffered on the commencement of the attack. As the violence of the disease
abates, a more generous diet may be adopted. If
the application of cold or exercise be not sufficient
to procure sleep, five grains of Extract. hyosciami, or
from fifteen to twenty drops of Tinct. digitalis, may
be taken at bed-time with advantage, during any
stage of the disease. I have also found the following draught very useful in these cases:—R. Mistur.
camphor. 1 oz. Liq. ammon. acet. 2 dr. Tinct. digitalis, 15 minims. Tinct. hyosciam. ½ dr. Syr. balsam.
1 dr.—Mix. But we scarcely possess any remedy
so generally powerful in allaying irritation as the
warm bath; there are very few persons, indeed,
upon whom it has not a salutary effect. It may be
used with advantage two or three times a week, or
even every day, if necessary: it is often found very
salutary to apply cold to the head when the patient
is in the warm bath. Whilst these remedies are
administered for the purpose of decreasing the diseased action of the brain, the requisite means must

be used to restore the other functions to their due tone. When, from the furred state of the tongue, and other symptoms, there is reason to conclude that the stomach is foul, I find that the quickest mode of obtaining relief is by giving an emetic: for, notwithstanding the use of them would appear contra-indicated from the act of vomiting propelling the blood to the head, I find this temporary inconvenience more than counterbalanced by the removal from that viscus of any irritating matter which, during its continuance, constantly tends to keep up the disease. And if, instead of emptying the stomach of the irritating matter at once by an emetic, we attempt to attain the same result by the slower method of purgatives and alteratives, we necessarily lose time. The diseased action of the brain and nervous system re-acts upon the viscera, and, in many cases, renders it a long and tedious process to restore these to a healthy state. Some judgment is required in determining the proper doses. In many cases, whilst the excess of circulation in the brain continues, it seems to absorb all the nervous and vital energy. The liver ceases to perform its functions aright, the patient will not discharge more than half a pint of urine in the course of the twenty-four hours, and in many cases the bowels are torpid, and there is no evacuation for several days. Now it is essential that all the functions should be restored to a healthy, but not to an excessive action. If very large doses of medicine be administered, there is

great risk that the viscera will be roused to excessive
and debilitating action for a time, and then will subsequently sink into a corresponding state of torpor.
The safest course is to give small, but repeated
doses ; but, if necessary, these must be increased until
the end is attained.   In many instances, after careful
perseverance in administering small and gradually
increased doses of the usual purgatives, it is found
requisite to have recourse to croton oil, in doses of
from one to two drops, repeated every four or six
hours, in order to get the bowels freely opened.
In other instances very small doses of cathartics are
sufficient.   But purgatives ought not to be administered when the secretions of the bowels are in a
healthy state, or in greater doses than are required
to keep them tolerably open.   It ought to be
observed, that in proportion as the diseased action
of the brain ceases, the bowels and other viscera
become more easily acted upon.   In cases where
the patients are plethoric, neutral salts generally
form the best purgatives : where the circulation is
deficient, or the digestive organs much impaired,
calomel, combined with the aromatic pill, is to be preferred.   But the same circumstances which indicate
the medicine proper to be selected in ordinary cases
are also the guide in cases of insanity.   The medical
attendant himself ought to inspect the egesta.   Very
little reliance can be placed on servants ; and the
patients are frequently so unable or unwilling to
describe their own feelings, that the state of the

body is the only guide as to the general health, and as to the proper mode of treatment. I have found the following prescription very useful in cases where the urinary secretions seem deficient ; and also in cases where it has been requisite to reduce the circulation :—Tinct. digital., Tinct. scillæ, aa. ½ oz., Vin antim. tart., Sp. æther. nitr. aa. 1 oz.—Mix. I usually administer it in doses of thirty drops three or four times a day, combined with ten grains of nitre. I would add, as a caution, that in every stage of insanity, great attention ought to be paid to the state of the skin : and when it is hot and dry, and the secretions deficient in quantity, five-grain doses of nitre, with a quarter or an eighth of a grain of tartar emetic, and a little sugar, ought to be administered every four hours. If the biliary secretions are also deficient, doses of two grains of pulv. antimonialis, with half a grain of calomel, may be substituted with advantage for the nitre and tartar emetic. It will be seen, that, in what has been said on the treatment of insanity, the division into mania and melancholia has not been observed. I am aware that they are usually considered as distinct diseases, requiring totally different modes of medical treatment. In the former, profuse bleedings and violent purgings are generally used : from this practice it will have been seen that I dissent entirely, except in the cases where the insanity has arisen from physical causes. In the latter, in the very early stage of the disease,

stimulants and tonics are generally administered.
Now, as far as I am capable of judging, mania and
melancholia both arise from an excess of blood,
although in different parts of the brain, and consequently a similar medical treatment is applicable
to both. I have certainly found cases of melancholia derive as much relief from cold applications
and repeated local bleedings, as cases of mania; and
I have no hesitation in saying, that a melancholic
patient will *ceteris paribus* bear as much depletion,
without injury to the constitution, as the maniacal
one.   When febrile action exists, nitre, antimony,
and other febrifuges, must be equally administered
to both.   These observations, with respect to blood-
letting, must be understood as entirely confined to
those cases where no phrenitis exists.   In cases of
phrenitis, immediate recourse must be had to very
copious bleedings from the system, from a large
orifice, and local bleedings will generally be found
to be subsequently necessary.   In cases of mania,
we find the violence of the patient and the quickness of the pulse greatly reduced by doses of sulphate of magnesia, with half a grain of tartar emetic
every three hours, until copious vomiting and stools
have been produced.   Small nauseating doses of
tartar emetic may also be applied with advantage
in the early stages of melancholia; and even in
those cases where the stomach appears to be out
of order, and the patient seems to have lost his
appetite and relish for food.   They diminish the

circulation in the brain, and by their temporary
relief enable it in some measure to recover its tone.
And certainly whilst the patient is suffering from
nausea, the most painful circumstances seem to produce but little effect on the mind; the feeling of
sickness absorbs every other consideration; and
any thing which tends to break in upon the habit
of constantly dwelling upon painful subjects, even if
it be but for a short time, is most valuable.   Cases
of melancholia are generally acknowledged to be
more difficult of cure than cases of mania.   This, I
think, arises from the circumstance, that in cases of
mania, the violence of the patient's conduct attracts
instant attention, and remedies are applied without
delay; whilst in melancholia, on the contrary, particularly when the disease arises from moral causes,
the alteration in the conduct and sentiments is so
gradual, that no notice is taken of it; and no
remedies are applied until the diseased action has
existed for a considerable period, and probably not
until diseased organization has actually taken place.
One of the first symptoms of the diseased action
of the brain having ceased, and of the secretions
having become natural, is the return of plumpness.
A detailed account of the particular medicines and
treatment, adopted in a number of cases, would
convey no useful information.   If the principles of
the treatment be rightly understood, the peculiar
constitution and circumstances of each patient will
be the best guide; and if they be not understood, it

would be perfectly in vain to hope that a transcript
of cases would make them intelligible.   In the
previous parts of the work, the effect of the general
plan in a variety of instances has been mentioned.
I have here inserted the short medical history of
two cases, as a specimen of what may be expected
as the ordinary result of the practice.   I have
added another, to show the propriety of using small
doses, especially of digitalis; and a fourth, to exemplify the state to which the chylopoietic viscera are
sometimes reduced, particularly after the disease has
not been properly attended to on its first appearance.

A. B., a female, about sixty-five years of age, had
been insane only a few weeks, and was in a state of
great agitation when admitted : head hot ; tongue
foul; bowels confined ; pulse one hundred and
twenty, and full.   Head was shaved, leeches applied,
an emetic and purgatives administered, and the
nitrate of potash, with the digitalis, given every four
hours.   The pulse was reduced in frequency, and
the general secretions improved by these means ;
but the cerebral irritation and extreme heat in the
superior part of the head continuing unabated, it
was necessary twice to repeat the bleeding by
leeches ; and the cold lotion was continued for some
time before the heat and irritation were removed.
The necessary low diet, with these depleting means,
though the bleeding was only local, relieved her
very considerably.   The mind became gradually
more composed.   No relapse took place **after**

amendment began, and she recovered her health, mental and bodily, in a few weeks, and was discharged cured.

J. S., a foreigner, was found in the street in a furious state of mania, and sent to the asylum as a lunatic vagrant.   Head hot, particularly in the region of the temples; extremities cold; tongue furred.   The head was ordered to be shaved, and kept cool with cold lotion, the extremities kept warm, and the bowels opened with calomel and ext. colocynth ; cupping-glasses were applied to the temples, and a blister to the back of the neck.   Ten grains of nitre, with thirty drops of the following prescription :—Tinct. digital., Tinct. scillæ, $\overline{aa}$. 2 dr., Sp. æther. nitr., Vin antim. tart. $\overline{aa}$. $\frac{1}{2}$ oz.— Mix,—given three times a day.   The powers of his mind and body were gradually restored.

This plan was continued, but with little improvement, for fourteen days.   Another blister was then applied to the back of the neck, and the calomel and the colocynth were repeated, but the drops were omitted; as the patient was thinner and much reduced in strength, and some small ulcers had appeared in the lower extremities indicating general debility, and the excessive heat in the head had abated.   A more nutritious diet was given ; the patient took a grain of sulphate of quinine three times a day ; and, as he continued to be restless at night, five grains of extract of hyoscyamus were given at bed-time ; the patient slept better, but was still mischievous, and sometimes dirty. This plan was persevered in, and the heat of the head and maniacal symptoms gradually abated. It soon became unnecessary to continue the hyoscyamus; and, by way of strengthening the general health and constitution, the shower-bath was ordered. The powers of his mind and body were gradually restored, and he returned quite well to his native country, in four months from the commencement of the attack. In this case, the only mode of ascertaining the state of the patient was from his bodily symptoms; as he could scarcely speak a word of any language except Polish.

T. L., reported to have been insane only a short time. Head hot, and complains of pain at the top of it; tongue white, and furred; pulse eighty-six, and full; bowels costive; mind much excited and wild. Head was ordered to be shaved, and afterwards kept cool with the evaporating lotion, and the extremities warm; he took an emetic, and the bowels were opened by a solution of sulphate of magnesia, which was followed by the mixture, containing ten grains of nitre and thirty of the foregoing drops, in each dose, three times a day. Balm tea when thirsty. The emetic and purgatives operated freely. The cold application succeeded in rendering the head cool; and, consequently, leeches and cupping-glasses were not applied. The following day the feet were warm, the pulse soft, but he had passed a restless night: the common evaporating lotion was omitted, and cloths dipped in a solution of half a drachm of extract of hyoscyamus, in about a pint of water, were kept continually wrapped about the head, and the other remedies were continued.   In three days the symptoms abated, the pulse was reduced in frequency and fulness, and he slept better.   At the end of a week, under this treatment, the pulse was brought down to sixty; the tongue clean, bowels open. The remedies were discontinued.   The mind gradually became less excited, and he was allowed a more generous diet, and further medicine became unnecessary.   At the time of this being written, not more than sixteen days have elapsed since his admission ; and he is now walking about the ward, rapidly improving in mind and in general health. In this case it will be observed, that although only five drops of tincture of digitalis, in conjunction with the nitre, were given at a dose, and only repeated three times in the twenty-four hours, at the end of a week the pulse was reduced from eighty-six to sixty.   The change of the evaporating lotion to the solution of hyoscyamus was an experiment : I can form no opinion, as to whether this had, or not, any influence in producing the rapid amendment.

The following case will illustrate the theory, that when the brain is in a very great state of excitement the nervous energy is so deficient in other parts, that the functions are not performed in a healthy manner, and that it is sometimes requisite to use very powerful medicine to restore them to healthy action ; though the organs themselves have undergone no organic change, and are capable of resuming their functions, as soon as the irritable state of the brain is subdued.

A. B., fifty-five years of age, of very active and diligent habits, and of high moral and religious principles, was observed by his family, contrary to his usual habit, to become taciturn and gloomy in his manner, and to appear dissatisfied and discontented. His sleep was at first only disturbed, but at length he used to lie awake nearly the whole night. These circumstances did not create much alarm in his family, so long as he continued to attend to his business. The diseased action of the brain continuing, other organs began at length to sympathize with it : he lost his appetite, and became generally unwell. His medical attendant prescribed some aperient medicine, which he often refused to take, and consequently daily got worse : he confined himself almost entirely to his house, and, as the winter was approaching, to his room. He had been in this state for about four months when I first saw him. He was very much dejected, and was labouring under morbid religious feelings : he had become thin, and the bowels were habitually very costive; head hot ; pulse, about ninety. As he was very obstinate, and neither his family nor medical attendant had any influence over him, I

recommended his immediate removal to a distance
from home ; and prescribed leeches, cold applications to the head, calomel and extract of colocynth,
to purge him.   None of these things were administered or attended to : he continued getting worse
in every respect. Six weeks afterwards I was again
desired to see him ; the patient, in addition to his
other sufferings, was then complaining of numbness
in one of the limbs ; and exhibited other symptoms,
denoting such a fulness of blood in the head, as to
create considerable alarm.   The patient was then
removed from home ;—the head was shaved, and,
all the upper portion of it being very hot, was bled
with leeches, and the evaporating lotion applied.
The secretions from the bowels and kidneys were
very deficient ; calomel and colocynth were given in
powerful doses without producing any effect ; and it
was necessary not only to repeat the pills, but to
give castor oil, sulphate of magnesia, enemas, and,
lastly, the croton oil in two-drop doses, before
any evacuation could be obtained.   The same difficulty was found with the kidneys ; not more than
half a pint of urine was obtained, sometimes, in
twenty-four hours. Diuretics combined with neutral
salts, in conjunction with extract taraxaci and pil.
hydrarg. were had recourse to, and the obstruction
was overcome.   Firm, but kind treatment con-
quered the self-will of the patient ; and, by degrees,
not only was he got down stairs daily, but was
induced to walk in the open air.   The tongue, as

might be expected, was generally furred; the pulse between ninety and a hundred, and the appetite deficient : the head also continued hot; it was necessary to keep it constantly cool with the evaporating lotion, and repeat the local bleeding. But it was not until several weeks elapsed, and the cerebral excitement had evidently abated, that any improvement was observed in the secretions : unusually large doses of purgatives were constantly required to keep the bowels open, and the diuretics to be continued to keep the urinary organs active. Steadily pursuing this plan, the pulse, after some weeks, began to abate in frequency; the tongue became cleaner, and the head cooler. In proportion as the cerebral irritation abated, the nervous system in general was restored to its equilibrium, the chylopoietic viscera were more easily acted upon, until the functions were performed without the aid of medicine. The patient, at the end of three months, was sufficiently recovered to take a journey into the country.

Although the plan of medical treatment previously pointed out is the best with which I am acquainted, for relieving the irritability attendant upon incipient insanity, and upon the exacerbations in old cases, yet there are many instances in which its operation, to say the least, is slow and uncertain. Local bleedings at the time appear to afford relief; but this seems to be rather the result of their removing from the brain the injury caused by irritation, than of their directly affecting and diminishing this irritation. I have very little doubt that there is in nature some medicine, with which I am at present unacquainted, that would operate as a specific in these cases. What it is, I know not; but it certainly is not to be found in any of the vegetable poisons in general use. I have seen them tried repeatedly; but whatever else may have been their effect, they do not seem specifically to act upon nervous irritability, although, as must have been already seen, some of them may be very generally used with advantage.

Let us next proceed to consider the moral treatment. The first object to be attained is, if possible, to remove the exciting cause of the disease. There are some cases, in which this may be effected without much difficulty. When the insanity has arisen from the actual presence of some objects, which operate too powerfully on the brain, the immediate removal to other scenes, with proper medical treatment, will prevent the increase of the attack, and speedily restore the patient. One of the persons, who came as a domestic to the institution at Hanwell, felt his mind so much excited by the presence of the patients, that he lost all appetite; he could obtain no refreshing sleep, and, in fact, could not close his eyes without having images of the patients continually dancing before him. There is no doubt that if he had remained in the institution, he would have become insane. His removal into other scenes, with proper medical treatment, soon restored him to his usual health. But unfortunately, in most instances, when the insanity arises from moral causes, the mind busies itself about some painful reality, which it is not in the power of the physician to remove; or it occupies itself too intensely about some subjects of sufficient real importance to engross all its attention. In the former instances, although the cause is rarely in the power of the physician, or even of the friends of the patient, yet, if from any circumstances it be removed, an attack may be prevented, or, if it have already supervened, one grand difficulty in the recovery of the patient will be overcome. It has been already stated, that pecuniary embarrassments are a fertile cause of insanity in England. It cannot be a matter of surprise that this should be the result in a country where speculation is carried on to so ruinous an extent, and where a delay in expected payments may reduce a man from affluence to poverty. One instance has occurred within my own observation, where relief from extreme embarrassment, with a little medical assistance, was sufficient almost immediately to restore the patient to health. A merchant, who had formerly carried on a very extensive business, from a series of losses became much reduced; he bore up against them, and struggled to support a wife and a large family, until he was induced foolishly to attempt to increase his capital by bill-drawing. This, as is usually the case, led to ruin. He was arrested and sent to prison, his little property was sold, and no resource but the work-house seemed left for him. He was a man of keen feelings. His intense anxiety, as might reasonably have been expected, brought on watchfulness and the usual symptoms of incipient insanity. As soon as his principal creditor became acquainted with the true state of the case, he had compassion upon him and released him from prison ; and one of his sons, a most amiable young man, who was in a good situation as a clerk, undertook to provide for the immediate wants of the family. The result was, that the health of the patient was speedily restored, and the attack of insanity, which was evidently coming on previously to his leaving the prison, was averted. But in those cases where the over-action of the brain has been brought on by thinking too long and too intensely on painful truths, from which there is no escape for the patient, it is exceed-ingly difficult to divert the attention, and to prevent the mind from dwelling upon them so conti-nually as to produce disease ; for although patients are conscious of the injury they are inflicting upon themselves, and of the inutility of their over-anxiety, and judge most accurately of their situations, they do not appear to possess the power of controlling their thoughts. In fact, the habit of severe mental discipline is too much neglected. If in ordinary circumstances, as a part of self-education, we were to accustom ourselves to fix certain limited times, on which to occupy the mind on particular subjects, to the exclusion of all others, and during those periods rigidly to confine the attention, and at the conclusion of them, carefully to change the current of our thoughts, we should obtain an habitual power over ourselves, which would be a most useful preservative against the over-anxiously dwelling upon painful subjects.   When the exciting cause cannot be removed, the patient should be placed in circumstances calculated as much as possible to produce a complete interruption to the train of thought; every object at all likely by association to recall to the mind the painful circumstances, should be avoided; the patient ought to be surrounded with other objects.   The usual routine of his habits ought to be broken in upon, and the attention attracted by a change in the little domestic arrangements; and, however painful, he should be at once withdrawn from the society of his friends.   If the diseased action be but small, and the attack just in its commencement, I know of no means of accomplishing this more effectually than by sending the patient on an excursion into a fine country, mountainous if possible: the air, the scenery, and the exercise, all have a salutary influence; and the separation is by this means effected without causing any pain either to him or to his friends; but he ought, if possible, to be accompanied during the journey, by an experienced medical attendant; and the physical remedies for the relief of the brain ought to be most

carefully attended to.   Much disappointment frequently arises from change of scene producing no
benefit.   This is to be traced to the neglect of the
use of medical remedies at the same time.   It would
not be less unreasonable to expect that inflammatory
action of the lungs, produced by cold, would be
cured by the mere removal into a warmer temperature, than to hope that the diseased action in
the brain should be cured merely by withdrawing
the patient from the immediate influence of the
cause of it.   Much mischief has arisen from this
mistake, and valuable time has been lost, to the
irreparable injury of the patient.   I know an
instance of a gentleman, who became insane, and
whose insanity was principally exhibited in general
depression of mind, and in erroneous views on
religious subjects.   His conduct was not such as to
make personal restraint necessary; and it was
thought that a journey on the continent would
divert the attention to other objects, and speedily
restore the mind.   This was tried; but medical
remedies being neglected, the result was such as
might have been feared.   The diseased action
increased, and he will in all probability be insane
for life.   When change of scene is tried, I should
strongly recommend varied excursions in a fine
country, and not the mere change of a residence in
a foreign capital.

If the diseased action exists to such an extent as
to make the change of scene inexpedient, or the

circumstances of the patient will not permit such a means of recovery to be resorted to, he ought to be at once removed from home, and placed under medical care. It is painful for friends to intrust their dearest relatives to strangers, and to run the risk on their recovery of being thought to have acted towards them harshly and precipitately; but unless they are willing to have the best interests of the sufferers sacrificed to a selfish caution and a foolish delicacy, they will not hesitate, however trying, to incur the responsibility of placing them, on the very commencement of the disease, where they will have an opportunity of receiving the best medical and moral treatment; and where they will at least be prevented from inflicting upon them-selves, or those about them, any bodily injury. Many valuable lives have been lost from a foolish delay in the adopting this decisive but necessary step.   In still more numerous instances, persons have remained insane for life, who, had promptness been used, might speedily have been restored to society.   County Lunatic Asylums offer to the poor the most efficient means of cure; and no induce-ment exists to keep them in confinement there a day longer than is desirable for their restoration and subsequent continuance in good health.   No such provision is at present within the reach of the wealthy; but the houses for the reception of the rich, and the asylums for the poor, are of so much importance, as to deserve more consideration

than could be conveniently given to them in
this place.

The first step on the part of the medical man, is
to gain the confidence of the patients by kind treatment, and a solicitude for their welfare. These are
soon perceived and properly appreciated. To engage their attention on some new object, either by
affording them useful employment or attractive
recreation, is the next step to be pursued. But
before any of the faculties of the mind which have
been in a diseased state are again called into
action, great care should be taken to ascertain that
no inflammation, or even irritation of the brain
remains. For though we well know that nothing
tends to the restoration of a weakened brain, or of
a weakened limb, so much as moderate exercise;
yet, if that exercise be commenced too soon, much
mischief is often the result. As this is an error into
which I have frequently fallen, I think it the more
necessary to caution others. So long as any symptoms of excessive circulation in the brain remain,
patients ought not to be permitted to use much exercise. They should be kept as quiet as possible until
these symptoms are removed by the medical treatment previously pointed out. In many cases, particularly amongst the industrious poor, whose previous
habits have rendered such a system of quiet, and an
abstinence from muscular labour irksome, a desire
is frequently expressed to be permitted to work
before the exercise would be prudent. But with

others of this rank, it is a task of no ordinary
difficulty to rouse the patients to any species of
exertion, mental or bodily.   This is particularly the
case where the disease has been of long standing;
the mind having become habituated to one train of
thinking, and the body to indolence, the greatest
repugnance to any exertion is felt.   In some constitutions nothing but the most determined perseverance can overcome it.   The great means of
accomplishing this, or indeed, of influencing the
conduct of the patients in any other respect, is by
ascertaining what they particularly like and dislike,
and then granting or withholding the indulgence,
according to their behaviour.   Very few persons
arrive at the period of life at which insanity comes
on without having acquired certain tastes and habits.
It is of the greatest importance that these should be
ascertained in each individual patient.   They are
the lever, and frequently the only lever, by which
the moral man can be moved.   When the bodily
health is restored, any little things which the patient
really enjoys should be withheld, and only granted
upon his complying with certain conditions, and
withdrawn on their being broken.   The medical
attendant ought to be ingenious in finding out the
peculiarities, and to be firm and kind in the treatment which he founds upon them.   He ought fully
to explain to the patient the reasons for his conduct
to him; and endeavour to impress upon the mind,
that any other mode of treatment would be a breach

of duty on his part, and that the deprivation is painful to him, but essential to the patient. In many cases, where the total indifference of a patient prevents this mode of treatment being used, the breaking in upon his habits has a similar effect.

A female, discharged as incurable from an hospital near London, was, on her admission into the asylum at Hanwell, one of the most distressing patients amongst the six hundred. The wringing of her hands, and her constant moaning, almost night and day, rendered her unfit to be amongst the other patients. Liberty and confinement, indulgence and privation were tried without effect; she still persevered in the deplorable noise and wringing of her hands. As she seemed to dislike the open air, she was ordered to be taken out of doors every morning, and there kept the whole day. For a long time no alteration seemed to take place; but the plan was still continued. In about two months her bodily health had greatly improved; and, although she refused to work, her noise was diminished, and she expressed her dislike of the going out of doors. This was a great point gained. She was told, that if she would conduct herself so as not to annoy the other patients, and amuse herself with a little work, she should remain in the house. On the promise of good behaviour, the experiment was tried, and it succeeded. She has, for weeks, daily occupied herself in sewing. She has little indulgences, the fruits of her labour; and she rarely attempts to wring her hands or to repeat her moaning : when she does, a hint that she must be removed from her nurse—to whom she is much attached—and again sent into the garden, is quite sufficient to recall her to order.   But it is impossible to point out the various modes of acting, according to this principle, on the minds of the patients.   They are as diversified as the temperaments, dispositions, and habits of each individual. An account of the various species of employment adopted at the asylum at Hanwell, and of the means practically used to engage the attention of the patients in them, will be given in a subsequent chapter.   Considerable tact is required in adapting the particular kind of occupation to the tastes of the patients.   They are usually more easily induced to work at the trades to which they have been brought up, than to turn their attention to pursuits entirely new.   Most men seem to have a natural fondness for farming and gardening, and these occupations have this great advantage, that there are certain portions of the labour in them, in which a violent or suicidal patient may be employed, without being entrusted with any tools by which he might either injure himself or others.   But so important do I consider the diverting the mind by employment, that where the patient cannot be induced thus to occupy himself, or where the occupation is too mechanical to keep the mind interested, I do not hesitate, with proper precautions, to intrust him with tools, even where

an inclination to suicide or to violence exists.   And
although I have adopted this plan in numbers of
cases, no accident has yet ensued, and it has frequently been the means of the patient's complete
recovery.   I will mention one instance.   A carpenter was admitted as a patient into the asylum
at Wakefield.   He had previously made several
attempts at self-destruction, and was then in a very
desponding state.   After the diseased action had
subsided, great dejection still remained; he was,
however, placed under the care of the gardener,
who was then constructing a kind of grotto or
moss-house in the grounds.   The contriving the
building offered a scope for his taste and ingenuity.
He was consulted on the arrangement of the floor,
which was formed of pieces of wood of different
kinds, set in various figures.   He was furnished
with tools, though he was, of course, most carefully
watched.   He took so great an interest in the
little building, that the current of his thoughts was
changed.   All his miseries were forgotten, and his
recovery took place at the end of a few months.
He very justly attributed his restoration to the
" moss-house."   Violent patients may frequently be
employed with tools, and with safety, by setting
them to work in a place entirely detached from the
others, or with one very quiet and harmless patient.
The great danger arises from allowing two or more
violent patients to be near each other.   It rarely
happens that a good-tempered, inoffensive person,

who does not attempt to interfere with them, or to control them, is injured.

As might reasonably be expected, from their previous habits, a much greater difficulty exists in inducing persons of higher rank to employ themselves in bodily labour, than those of the lower classes. But there is something so congenial to the natural tastes of men in the cultivation of the ground, that with a little management and address, many who have been solely accustomed to mental exertion may easily be persuaded to busy themselves out of doors. This is exceedingly beneficial; for, in addition to the moral advantage derived from the mind being diverted, there is an actual physical good, by the exercise turning the blood and vital energy to the supply of muscular power, and preventing excess of circulation in the internal organs. Of course, many will be found to whom such an employment would be irksome; but, whatever be the rank of life, or the difference in outward circumstance, man is still the same being. He feels pain when deprived of the comforts which he has been in the habit of enjoying;—he is to be won by kindness, and he is offended at harshness or want of courtesy. The being excluded from the society of all whose good opinion is valued, begets in the insane, as it would tend to do in the sane, a habit of giving utterance to momentary feelings, without considering their propriety. And with both, where the mind has no opportunity of employment on objects of importance, it will either busy itself about trifles, or sink into apathy, or allow itself to wander unchecked in idle reveries. In Hogarth's picture of Bedlam, the straw crown was not the mere symbol of madness; the making it, however valueless, tended to the happiness of the patient, and was an act of practical wisdom. It was, in fact, the result of the same feeling which induced the lonely prisoner to make companions of the spiders in his dungeon. Now what would be the consequence if we were to take a sane person, who had been accustomed to enjoy society, and to have " space for his horses, equipage, and hounds," and were to lock him up in a small house, with a keeper for his only associate, and no place for exercise but a miserable garden? We should certainly not look for any improvement in his moral and intellectual condition. Can we then reasonably expect, that a treatment which would be injurious to a sane mind, should tend to restore a diseased one? But, unfortunately, this is the plan too generally adopted with the rich, both males and females.

A young lady possesses great natural abilities, high accomplishments, and considerable personal attractions. She receives the attention and admiration of society. She marries early in life, and employs her time and talents, as is usual among persons of fashion, in giving and receiving pleasure. Adverse circumstances, jealousy, or other moral causes, bring on insanity. The disease assumes a maniacal form. The usual routine of treatment is adopted without any permanent improvement: after the lancet, cathartics, and blisters, have been vigorously used, she is sent to a private house, and placed under the care—very possibly—of kind-hearted persons, who do all in their power to abate the violence of the paroxysm. In a shorter or longer time the disease begins to wear itself out. From its violence having rendered personal restraint necessary, one or two stout women are selected to take charge of her. In such cases, the patient usually has her private apartments, to which no other patients are admitted. It is therefore more than probable that she has no other society than that of her attendants, whose manners are totally at variance with all her previous habits. She soon becomes familiarized with every object in the house and garden ; and, as there is nothing to divert her attention, her mind naturally continues to brood over the melancholy subject, which has been the cause of her insanity. Under these circumstances but little prospect of cure exists. The various feelings and faculties of the mind, which if recalled to their former activity would banish the one absorbing idea, now lie dormant, from the absence of every object calculated to arouse them. Over-action and excess of circulation continue in a portion of the brain, until at length lesion ensues, and she becomes hopelessly and irrecoverably insane. This description accurately marks the progress of the disease in numerous instances.

In a well-regulated institution, every means ought to be invented for calling into exercise as many of the mental faculties as remain capable of employment. We must remember, that the happiness of man, whatever be his situation in life, consists in the proper and harmonious exercise of all his powers, moral, mental, and physical. Insanity, brought on from moral causes, is the result of too great and partial exercise of some of the feelings or faculties ; the patient, therefore, ought to be surrounded with objects calculated to attract attention, and to divert the mind from the contemplation of its sufferings. In those cases where vicious pursuits have previously occupied the time, the salutary restraint from them will render the mind susceptible of pleasure from innocent occupation. For persons in the higher ranks of society, a mansion should be provided, with park, woods, lawns, hot-houses, gardens, and green-houses. It should be fitted, internally, with every convenience and luxury for the gratification of the taste. Science and the fine arts ought to be pressed into the service of stimulating the dormant faculties to healthy exercise. There should be, as there is now at Aversa, a music-room, which the patients of both sexes should daily have the privilege of using ; and one evening in every week should be specially devoted to a dress-concert or oratorio, to which all, in a fit state to attend, should be invited. Such an association of patients, of the two sexes, would have a very happy influence on both. And an additional impetus should be given, by remunerating for their assistance any professional persons, either male or female, residing in the neighbourhood. This would enliven the evening's entertainment, and make it more valued. It would also tend to lead the feelings to a profitable contemplation of happier days, by showing that the capability and the means of enjoyment, in this respect at least, were left; and it might awaken the hope, that the avenues to other pleasures, moral and intellectual, might soon be opened. In a similar manner, scientific amusements should be cultivated ; one evening in each week should be devoted to them. Lectures on chemistry, with suitable apparatus for the performance of the minor experiments, would afford much entertainment; and this might easily be provided. An orrery should form an appendage. There should be a modelling-room, and a studio, where those who have a taste for the fine arts should have an opportunity of receiving weekly instruction. Botany ought to be sedulously cultivated; the open garden, the green-house, and the hot-house, would, according to taste, to power of exercise, and to the required warmth of constitution, afford important means of cure, both moral and medical. The various domestic animals and birds, with others of rarer species, would contribute to interest and amuse. The library should be well furnished ; but, of course, care and discrimination would be required in the selection of books, adapted to the particular habits, and to the states of mind of the patients. An appeal to the moral and benevolent feelings will arouse a patient from his morbid feeling to useful action, when a merely intellectual inducement is ineffectual. Point out the sufferings of the poor, either by a personal visit or by oral description, and show that it is in the power of the morbid-minded individuals, by their efforts, to relieve the wants or to add to the comforts of the afflicted; and many will cheerfully exert themselves, whom no other inducements would influence. The clothes for the expected baby will be made, and the comforts of the mother attended to. By both sexes uniting in a work of benevolence, more will be done, and with greater cheerfulness and benefit to the patients, than could be accomplished by their separate efforts. They will mutually stimulate each other; and if a promise be given on the part of a gentleman to contribute his share, the lady will take care that the good shall not fail from any backwardness on her part. The natural feeling of interest and kindness, generated in the mind towards those whom we have benefited, tends delightfully to counteract the morbid feelings existing among the insane. Those, who have strictly conscientious and religious feelings, afford another ground to work upon. Let them be induced to employ themselves in drawing, or in making any little articles, from which profit may be derived, and inform them that it will be applied for those religious or benevolent purposes in which they feel most interested, and there will be no lack of industry. The well-educated and the wealthy would cheerfully exert themselves for the destitute wanderer. There would then be an evidently useful object in their employment; and with the insane as well as with the sane, labour of every kind requires the stimulus of a prospective good. Few minds are so constituted as to be able to employ themselves merely from an abstract notion, that activity is conducive to happiness. One great error in dealing with the insane is in treating them as if they were differently constituted from the sane. They are frequently asked to work, without knowing for what purpose; and, as might be expected, such occupation becomes tedious, and is at length refused. Indeed such labour is as wearisome to an attendant as it is monotonous and uninteresting to the patient. But it is in vain to hope to rouse the intellectual and the nobler faculties of patients in the higher ranks, so long as they are left to the society of a keeper or a nurse. They ought to be the associated companions of persons of benevolent dispositions, of refined habits, and of cultivated tastes. And if asylums were conducted upon liberal and rational principles, there would be no lack of eligible competitors for the office. The young medical man would find a few months spent in such an institution, previous to his commencing practice, a most delightful means of general improvement; and the young lady, whose finances might require her to do something for her support, would have, in the gently winning back the suffering mind to reason and to happiness, full scope for her best and noblest faculties.   Indeed I should not consider that an asylum for the rich had attained its highest point of moral management, until it had become so happy a place of residence, that the patients when restored should regret the quitting it, unless drawn from it by ties of family and affection.   Were such retreats for the insane to exist, no more reluctance would be felt in sending the insane to an asylum for moral cure, than is now experienced in placing children at a school for discipline and instruction.

Many reasons exist which will sufficiently account for the fact, that no such a retreat for the insane is to be found.   In the first place, the capital which would be required to supply all the requisites would be such, as no individual would feel himself justified in expending, particularly as the prospect of his being ultimately repaid would depend almost entirely upon the continuance of his life, and of such a measure of health as would enable him to fulfil his professional duties.   But there is a still stronger reason; it is not to the interest of the proprietor of a private asylum to cure his patients.   In every other disease successful treatment raises the reputation, and tends to increase the practice of a professional man; and a patient when cured feels a pleasure in recommending to others the individual from whose assistance he has derived important benefit. But with those who have recovered from insanity, every circumstance which, in the most distant way, alludes to the affliction, is carefully avoided; and neither the patient nor the friends would be willing to have its previous existence suspected. And those whose friends are attacked, would think it almost an insult to make any inquiry even of the relatives of one who had recovered, as to the skill and kindness of the person under whose care he had been placed. Indeed they feel it a species of disgrace to be connected, although remotely, with any one capable of benefiting by such information. After the relative has been consigned to an asylum, in most instances his recovery soon ceases to be expected; and in many it is never desired. There is not, therefore, the same inducement to stimulate a professional man to careful and active exertion, to find out means of cure for this disease, which operates upon him in every other. But the evil goes still further. There are instances, and these not rare, and occurring too amongst the patients from whom the greatest emolument is derived, in which it is the direct and positive interest of the relative who has placed the patient in confinement, that he should never be restored to society; and without imputing improper motives either to the relative or to the medical man, we know that self-interest tends to bias the judgment, and that with great wealth with the one, and a permanent income with the other, depending upon the patient continuing insane, it is inconsistent with human nature to expect that the same anxious and unwearied care for his cure will be exhibited, as if a personal benefit were to accrue from his recovery. Although, under the present system of inspection, it would be difficult to retain a sane person long in an asylum; yet it is impossible to secure by it the diligent application of every medical and moral means of cure, with the careful avoiding of every circumstance, however minute, which would tend to cause irritation. I do not mean to say that there are not many amongst my professional brethren, whose high sense of rectitude does not overcome the evils resulting from the system. But men are unhappily placed, where their duty is continually at variance with their interest. It is exceedingly difficult to suggest any means of avoiding this. In fact, when a man becomes insane, he is entirely at the mercy of his friends; and when self-interest has banished affection from their bosoms, it is impossible to make any provision, which will secure to him that watchful attention to his welfare, for which he must from necessity be indebted to them. I am quite incapable of suggesting any means of relief for one, who, in consequence of being retained at home, or placed in a house with no other insane person, is out of the reach of inspection. But still, much would be done if an asylum were provided upon such a plan as would furnish all appliances for cure, and were placed under the direction of one, who should derive no benefit by the patients remaining in it, but who would feel his professional reputation interested in their recovery.   It is true, that in some of the county asylums, patients of the higher classes are admitted, and that in these there is no temptation improperly to retain them ; but a great objection is felt on the part of the friends to allow their relatives to be in an asylum with paupers ; and in many of these institutions, the subscribers residing in the neighbourhood, both ladies and gentlemen, are formed into a numerous and constantly changing body of visitors.   This is quite sufficient to prevent persons of the higher classes sending their relatives to such institutions ; indeed nothing can be more prejudicial to the patients, than to be exposed to the magisterial visits of those with whom they have been in the habit of associating : and on their recovery, the meeting, in the daily intercourse of society, the witnesses of their sufferings and degradation, is most painful and humiliating, particularly to persons of the higher rank. A man, under these circumstances, feels his self-respect lessened, and he cannot meet his fellow-man on equal terms.   It is an evil to which the poor are not exposed, as the visitors are not taken from the class of their companions. This system also tends to cramp the energies of the superintendent.   When his best efforts for the welfare of his patients are liable to be misunderstood, and thwarted by a visitor, whose annual subscription has given him, during his monthly rotation, the power, but not the requisite knowledge, to interfere, he gradually ceases to exert himself, and is content with kindly performing a dull routine of uninteresting duties.

Another error is of frequent occurrence in the management of county asylums. The medical superintendent and matron, who live on the spot, and are nominally at the head of the institution, have really very little discretionary power. One or two of the physicians residing in the neighbourhood, and who are expected to visit the patients once or twice a week, have, in many of them, the entire direction ; the superintendent and matron having little more to do, than to carry their orders into execution. The necessary result is, that there is a division of responsibility. The superintendent, finding himself a mere agent, becomes indifferent to the success of the institution ; and the physician being incapable, during his medical visits, of organizing the details (although these materially affect the patient), does not feel himself responsible for the domestic or moral management. Now it is not possible that an asylum can be well conducted, unless those who are on the spot are most zealously alive to every little thing which can, by possibility, contribute to the well-being of the patients. It is by the multiplicity of these little things that great effects are produced.

The dispositions, habits, and temperaments of the individual patients, must be watched from day to day; and the moral treatment, and, in a great measure, the medical also, must be adapted and varied, according to the peculiar and changing circumstances of each. Now no person ought to be appointed as the resident medical superintendent who is not (no matter whether he be physician, surgeon, or apothecary,) medically and morally qualified for the office: and if he be so qualified he will, from being constantly on the spot, have much greater opportunities of observing the peculiarities of the patients, and of making himself familiar with every turn of the disease, and the treatment required for it, than a medical man who only pays short and occasional visits to the institution; and he will have the still further stimulus for his exertions, of knowing that his reputation is at stake in their success. With honourable and high-minded men, (and no others ought to be selected,) this will be of more avail than a code of regulations, and a regiment of visitors to put them in force. It is a foolish economy not to offer a sufficient remuneration, to induce men of the first respectability in the profession, to be candidates for such situations. Of course, cases will occur, in which the most skilful man may desire additional assistance. Let him have the privilege of calling in, when he finds it necessary, the advice of a consulting physician: this will suggest to him new remedies, or increase his confidence in the course he is adopting, without lessening his responsibility. At present, the county asylums are not an adequate provision for the reception of the higher classes, and very few of the higher classes are to be found in them.

Indeed I am not acquainted with one, at all coming up to my notions of what an asylum for the rich ought to be ; but I still think, that it is perfectly practicable to provide for them an institution, possessing every means for cure, and every requisite for their comfort and happiness, combined with but little risk of their being improperly detained. I should recommend an asylum on the same principle as the Proprietary Schools. Let a number of gentlemen subscribe, in shares, a sufficient capital for the purpose ;—let a committee of management be selected; a proper house, grounds, furniture, and apparatus be procured, and the rates of admission determined by the committee, who would, of course, have the power of refusing any applications. A resident medical superintendent should be appointed, who should have a fixed salary, and should not be allowed to derive the slightest pecuniary benefit from the patients remaining in the house. The medical and moral treatment should be under his direction, and his certificate of a patient's fitness for discharge, should be final and decisive. The costs of such an establishment would not be so great as might at first be supposed. It would be unnecessary to erect a building expressly for the purpose. A large mansion, which might be purchased for a comparatively small sum, might easily be converted into such an establishment. As it is quite obvious, that although the disease is the same in the rich as in the poor, many of the expensive contrivances which are required for paupers would be unnecessary, where each attendant has not under his charge more than one or two patients : for instance, airing courts, with their walls, which are essential where there is only one keeper to twenty or thirty patients, would be worse than useless in such an institution. The grounds must be the airing courts, and the vigilance of the attendants must supply the place of walls. The whole establishment should resemble, as much as possible, an ordinary habitation. The usual living rooms should present no appearance of confinement, though in these the windows may easily be prevented from opening beyond a certain height. Apartments must be provided, properly secured and fitted up with shutters and wire blinds, where the patients may be removed during violent paroxysms : but very few of such rooms would be requisite. The great expense would be in the attendance, and in keeping up the gardens and pleasure-grounds, and in the providing horses and carriages, and other means, for the employment and recreation of the patients. But if the institution contained one hundred patients, the income would abundantly supply every want, and leave an ample profit to the shareholders. I am decidedly of opinion, that it would be greatly to the benefit of the patients, for the same establishment to contain both males and females : of course, there must be sufficient means not only of separation, but of entire exclusion, where it is desirable; but I am fully convinced, that the well-regulated association of the two sexes would exert a salutary moral influence on both. Of course, in such an institution wealth would, as elsewhere, procure for its possessor additional comforts : but the distinction should be there confined to the private accommodation of the patients. The rich man should, if his friends thought well, have his three or four rooms ; and these might be larger, and more splendidly fitted up, than those of his poorer neighbour. But, in the public association of the house, there should be no distinction between the man who contributed a thousand pounds, and the one who contributed a hundred pounds a year. The only rule of classification in the different sets of public rooms should be, according to the different states of the disease, and the various habits and education of the patients. I cannot but think that such an institution would be a blessing to society : it would afford to persons of the highest classes a means of cure, combined with the happy and rational exercise of their faculties. Instead of being shut up, companionless, in a small solitary dwelling, they would have cheerful association, with space and opportunity for every salutary employment and recreation. Nor would the middling classes be without their share in its benefit; although, from the want of means, they are at present generally exempt from that solitary confinement which is inflicted, as the greatest punishment, upon criminals, and administered, from mixed feelings of kindness and pride, to the rich insane; they still have not those advantages which this system would secure to them. By no other means could they, at the same moderate rate, participate in those comforts and elegancies which must, in such an establishment, be provided for the rich. If such an institution were to be formed, and placed under proper care, there would be no lack of patients. There ought to be at the head of it a medical man, well acquainted with the disease, of undoubted integrity, and of high moral and religious character; and, as an essential qualification, he ought to possess an active and much enduring benevolence. He should not be easily provoked, and he should have a sufficient genuine regard to his patients firmly to deny them any thing, however painful to himself, which he would know would be prejudicial to them; and rigidly and constantly to enforce, with unwearied watchfulness and diligence, every plan for their welfare. There should be associated with him, in the honourable task of winning back the wandering and perverse to reason and to happiness, one, who would be in every respect his helpmate for the undertaking.

She ought to be willing to sacrifice, at the shrine of humanity, every feeling of self-indulgence, and every prejudice of education and society; and although, from natural endowments and mental cultivation, she should excel in gently drawing out the sensitive and retiring mind, and in ingeniously mingling the cup of consolation, according to the peculiar woes of the sufferer; she should feel nothing beneath her notice, that could allay the pangs or promote the comfort of the poorest imbecile, though incapable of distinguishing his benefactress, or of repaying her kindness even with a look of gratitude. And she ought to have under her training a noble band of young and highly-gifted females, actuated by similar motives, and willing, from love to God and man, to assist her in her anxious efforts. I am far from decrying the benefits to be derived from the exertions of my own sex, but I know from experience, that these are nothing, in comparison to the moral advantages to be gained by the benevolence and activity of woman. And it would be unjust in me if I did not acknowledge, that if I have met with any measure of success in my attempts to rouse the dormant faculties, to alleviate the sufferings of the insane, and to render the patients under my care a happy and a united family; this success is mainly to be attributed to the abilities, the courage, the perseverance, the kindness, and the engaging manners of my wife. The female mind possesses a quickness of perception, and a ready tact, which are of much more efficacy in winning upon the insane than all the slower, and more serious, business-like efforts of our sex. Indeed, both amongst the sane and the insane, when a new trade has been to be learnt, the women have acquired it with twice the facility of the men; and have expressed a pleasure in being taught, whilst the men have, generally speaking, gone to the work heavily and unwillingly; and have only been induced to persevere from the hope of reward, or from being ashamed at the more rapid progress of the females. And in commencing any new manufacture together, the particular portion of the work which has required the greatest skill has been uniformly allotted to the women; and, after they have learnt it, the men have slowly and tediously been taught their lesson. In an asylum conducted upon the Proprietary principle, there would be every inducement for the medical superintendent to exert himself to the uttermost for the recovery of his patient; and, if he had at his disposal the means and the assistance previously pointed out, the majority would be speedily restored.

In many cases, the dissipated and vicious would learn, in such an institution, the practical happiness of religion and self-government, and would leave it useful and honourable members of society. In a large establishment, there would probably be some whose minds would be incapable of appreciating the value of a refined association, and whose wants could be adequately supplied by a kind and judicious nurse or keeper : but none ought to be considered to come under this class, until the most ingenious and persevering efforts had been made unsuccessfully to rouse every latent spark of mind and feeling. Much may be done by kindness and a scrupulous attention to the polite etiquette of society, even with those whose reason seems almost extinct. I know one instance, where, from continued confinement day and night for years, the limbs had become contracted, the fingers twisted over each other, and the patient totally insensible to the calls of nature. Two stout, ignorant servants, neither of whom could read or write, had been the constant attendants. The maniacal violence and impatience of restraint, with which the commencement of the disease was characterized, seemed to have banished from their minds every idea of treating the poor sufferer with decency or respect : and when the first violence of the attack had subsided, no solace was offered to the feelings of wounded pride; but a constant source of irritation remained, in the being obliged to submit to the domination of such associates. An airing was sometimes taken, though the miserable patient, tied hand and foot, was fastened in a blanket to the bottom of the chaise. No wonder that these circumstances should have produced their natural results, and that on an occasional visit from the friends, sufficient violence should have been found, as apparently to have made such severe confinement necessary. Even this case was not beyond the reach of amelioration. A removal into different society, kind, soothing, and respectful manners, the absence of all restraint, except during the actual continuance of the paroxysm, have rendered the patient cleanly, comparatively happy, and exempt from any exacerbation of the disease, for six weeks together. Careful friction of the limbs has restored the use of the muscles, and the patient now enjoys a walk or a ride untrammelled. If such be the results where the disease has been of so long continuance, and the mental faculties apparently destroyed, no case ought to be considered sufficiently desperate to warrant the intrusting the patient at once to the society of the keeper or the nurse, or the neglecting any means which may possibly tend to cure the disease, or to diminish the sufferings. I cannot forbear mentioning another instance, to show the importance of proper moral treatment and its powerful effects, even in cases of long standing. A person of great talents and strong feelings, who had been accustomed from early life to elegant and refined society, became insane from too anxious thought on religious subjects. The melancholy, which was the first symptom of the disease, was succeeded by great maniacal violence. The patient was taken from home, and was for several years generally kept under personal restraint; and during the whole of the time the society was either that of the immediate attendants, or of other insane persons. The passions were entirely without control; the language became abusive and violent, although there still remained a capability of giving rational answers to most questions. The constant confinement had caused paleness and emaciation. After this system had been continued for many years, the patient was placed where an opportunity was offered of the association of a cheerful and polite family circle, on the condition of good and proper behaviour; and an assurance was given, that personal restraint should not be resorted to, until violence of conduct rendered it absolutely necessary. A great change for the better could not be expected to take place immediately; but the first trial showed that the proper motives had been acted upon. An instant banishment to the private apartments, on the exhibition of any violation of the decorum of society, gradually superinduced a habit of self-control. There was not any occasion to use personal confinement; the temporary banishments from society became less and less frequent. In fact, the feelings seemed to be carefully pent up, until the retirement of the private room gave an opportunity of giving them vent, without incurring the penalty of the forfeiture of the social advantages. The patient became conscious when the feelings were becoming incapable of control, and voluntarily retired into the private apartment. These occasions gradually became less frequent, and, with the exception of particular attacks of insanity, when the room is still kept, no symptoms of violence, and very few even of derangement, are exhibited. Constant exercise in the open air has quite reinstated the bodily health.

In the moral treatment of cases of insanity, it is of great importance to ascertain the ruling passion of the patient: an appeal to this will frequently divert the attention, and obviate the necessity of having recourse to violent measures. A female, of great firmness, had for several days refused to take her food, and as no persuasion seemed to have any influence upon her, preparations were made to inject it by the stomach-pump. At this juncture my wife discovered that the woman had naturally a great love of acquiring. She sat down by the patient's bedside, and without saying any thing on the subject of food, conversed with her on her former habits; and having learnt that she had kept cows and poultry, she induced her to give an account of the profits she made by them. This attracted the attention of the woman: she forgot her determination to resist; and whilst talking of the gain of selling the butter, she permitted herself to be fed with a basin of bread and milk, apparently unconscious that she was submitting to the wishes of her attendants. In this instance phrenology was of practical use. The existence of the strong feeling of love of gain was ascertained solely by the observation of the head at the time. Another instance of the power of checking the violent operation of one set of feelings by calling another into action, also occurred to my wife. A patient, who was pruning some trees in the garden, quarrelled with another lunatic, during the accidental absence of the gardener: he became so irritated that he threatened to kill the other. A third patient ran into the house to give the alarm. He met my wife on the way, and she returned with him to the combatants, and desiring to speak with the man who had the knife, told him she was surprised to find a man, of his talents and understanding, so far forgetting himself as to dispute with the other, who, as he knew, had been insane for several years. This gratified his self-esteem. He said, You are right, ma'am; I shall take no farther notice of him; —and he at once became quiet. It not unfrequently happens, that patients, of very irritable tempers, are suddenly thrown into violent paroxysms of passion from slight causes, and are as often to be diverted out of them, by calling other faculties into operation, by very simple methods. Many years ago, when the workmen were fitting up the asylum at Wakefield with gas-pipes, one of them carelessly left, in one of the wards, an iron chisel more than three feet long. A very powerful and violent patient seized it, and threatened to kill any one that should go near him. Keepers and patients all got out of his way, and he alone was soon in possession of the gallery, no one daring to go near him. After waiting a little time, until he was at the further end of it, I went towards him quite alone. I opened the door, and balancing the key of the ward on the back of my hand, walked very slowly towards him, looking intently upon it. His attention was immediately attracted ; he came towards me, and inquired what I was doing. I told him I was trying to balance the key, and said at the same time that he could not balance the chisel in the same way, on the back of his hand. He immediately placed it there ; and extending his hand with the chisel upon it, I took it off very quietly, and without making any comment. Though he seemed a little chagrined at having lost his weapon, he made no attempt to regain it, and in a short time the irritation passed away.

The "love of children" is another very powerful and general feeling, particularly amongst women. Great advantage may be taken of it, in diverting the mind from painful reflections. I have frequently known a patient, who has been for some time in a state of great excitement, become quite calm on the sight of a child, and amuse herself in attending to it for hours together. Indeed, where the love of children is strongly marked, conversation on the subject, judiciously timed, rarely fails to produce soothing and salutary results. It is impossible to account for the great effect occasionally produced in the minds of the insane by circumstances apparently most trivial. The result is beautifully given in the following lines :—

> " Oh, reason ! who shall say what spells renew,
>   When least we think of it, thy broken clew !
> Through what small vistas o'er the darken'd brain,
> Thy intellectual day-beam burst again ;
> And how, like forts, to which beleaguers win
> Unhoped-for entrance through some friend within,
> One clear idea waken'd in the breast
> By memory's magic, lets in all the rest."

A practical illustration occurred at Wakefield. H. R., a female about forty years of age, had been insane for some years when admitted. She was a very robust woman, and being usually in a state of excitement, was the terror of all the patients in the ward, when not in confinement. If at any time a softened influence could be produced upon her, and more gentle feelings called forth, it was by referring to the scenes of early life. One day, when under these impressions, a patient began a song, which she had learnt when a girl, when turning to my wife, who stood near her, she said with great anima- tion, " Mistress, when I was young I knew that song, and I think I could sing it now." She began, and, with the greatest delight, found she remem- bered the whole of it. From that hour " a change came o'er the spirit of her dream : " her excessive violence gave place to the more amiable and kindly feelings. Instead of being the dread of all about her, she became obliging and industrious. After some months of trial she got well and returned home. Some years afterwards she came over to pay us a visit, and at that period had had no return of the disease. The advantage of presence of mind and apparent confidence in the patients, when from circumstances placed in their power, during a paroxysm, was strikingly exemplified in the conduct of my wife towards this patient. In one of her most furious ebullitions of passion she contrived to seize her, and to twist her hand in her hair at the back of her head, and she looked at her with a countenance expressive of the utmost rage, and told her, that she could " twist her head round ;" which, from her great strength, was almost literally the truth : when my wife answered, with perfect calmness, " Yes, you could ; but I know you would not hurt a single hair." This confident appeal pacified her, and she immediately quitted her hold.

I hardly know whether it is right to appear to acknowledge the reality of the delusion in order to use it as a means of cure ; but this may occasionally be done, greatly to the advantage of the patient. A woman supposed that a witch besprinkled her face every night with cantharides : the impression was so strong, that for a long time she was gradually suffering in bodily health from want of sleep, as she passed the night in fighting the witches. A charm was pretended to be found out which would set all the witches at defiance. A little coloured milk was applied to the face, with a direction to keep the eyes closed, and to remain perfectly silent and quiet, as the whole efficacy of it would be broken by a single word being spoken, or the least motion being made. She was perfectly quiet during the night, and though she considered herself still under the influence of the witches, with the continued application of the milk she enjoyed undisturbed sleep, and her bodily health greatly improved.

Persons whose nervous temperament is obtuse, and who have none of that irritability which is so usually seen to exist amongst the insane, can scarcely conceive what very slight causes produce powerful moral effects upon them. A young woman, who had been but a short time insane, was brought to the asylum at Wakefield one evening, when nearly dark. The entrance to it was through a very large pair of wooden doors. Before a carriage could be driven into the front court, it was awkwardly enough arranged that it must go over an iron weighing-bridge: this, with the formidable appearance of the building, and the rumbling of the carriage upon the bridge, altogether produced such an effect upon the young woman, as that, to use her own words, "it turned her heart upside down." A great change certainly took place at the time, for she never exhibited any symptoms of insanity; and she herself attributed the alteration in her feelings to the kind of terror she then experienced.

The principle of fear may often be very successfully worked upon as a moral means of cure. When the patient is naturally timid, a dread of consequences will frequently induce self-control. The mere abstaining from extravagant conduct, and the ceasing to give utterance to violent expressions have a great tendency to diminish the irritation. This feeling is generally more easily worked upon by talking to others of the patients, in their presence, than by any direct threats. I remember the case of a poor girl whose constant moaning, during the night, disturbed the other patients. They requested that she might be removed from the ward. A representation, in her presence, of the exceedingly painful situation in which she must be placed, and of the very severe measures which must be adopted if she were removed, with a hope that the other patients would try her one night longer, produced such an effect upon her mind that, from fear of the consequences, she refrained from making the noise and laid still in bed. In a few nights the restraint she imposed upon herself produced sleep. She gradually became more and more tranquil, and eventually got quite well. But there are some cases, in which the mere threat, however conveyed, produces no salutary effect. It has already been stated that, in insanity, the evil dispositions which existed prior to the coming on of the disease still remain; and many of these are excited to increased action by the general irritability produced by it. It is always, therefore, a matter of great consequence to determine whether the conduct is the result of moral evil, naturally inherent in the man, or whether it arises from insanity ; that is, from diseased action of any particular part of the brain. Much of the moral treatment depends upon this ; for though it would be most cruel to subject the patient to any discipline, either moral or physical, for conduct arising from the latter, yet, as part of what is objectionable arises from the former, no little watchfulness is required to keep in check evil passions, frequently long indulged without any restraint. Happily the whip has for some time, at least in this country, ceased to be allowed in any Lunatic Asylum; and the more humane and rational plan of punishment, by deprivation and confinement, has been substituted in its place. It sometimes however happens, that patients are met with who are so obstinate and incorrigibly perverse, that these means alone are not sufficient. The shock of the electrifying-machine, which is often found beneficial in cases where the powers want rousing, is, in cases of determined obstinacy and bad conduct, equally useful. The terror of the machine will often overcome the vicious inclination. The same effect is frequently produced by the shower-bath, but still more so by the use of the circular-swing. These, however, are remedies which should never be had recourse to until all other means have failed; and then, never without the most explicit orders from the medical superintendent, who ought to be present whenever the latter is applied. Under these restrictions the most beneficial results often ensue ; and patients soon learn to put themselves under that discipline which will exempt them from such uncomfortable consequences. By patient perseverance in kindness, with indulgence as a reward of good conduct, and great firmness in the application of the requisite means to overcome obstinacy and perverseness, many patients who, from faulty education, had never been taught to exercise any control over their passions, have gradually become quiet and orderly, and have been eventually restored to reason. Kind and judicious conversation is a powerful moral means of cure. In many cases, where it appears to be listened to with indifference, it is often attended to, and subsequently carefully pondered over ; and the mere act of thinking upon it diverts the mind, and gives a rest to the over-excited feelings. The patient frequently seems at once to make a great advance towards recovery. Sometimes the improvement continues, but no further change for the better is observed until another step seems suddenly to be gained ; and after a time, the patient will as rapidly appear to lose ground, until another favourable change takes place, and he gradually and slowly recovers. I have no doubt that many of the checks might be avoided if what was passing in the mind of the patient were better known. The most trifling expressions, a word, or even a look may produce painful workings of the mind, ill suited to the newly

excited action of the weakened brain. The conversation of the friends of the patients frequently tends
materially to retard their cure. In public institutions the natural anxiety of the friends to see the
patients is one of the greatest difficulties to be contended with. In numerous instances patients, who
were apparently recovering very speedily, have been
thrown back nearly into the same state as on admission, merely from seeing their friends. The sight of
relatives recalls distressing associations to the mind;
and, too often, the well-meant but ill-timed information, of their being much wanted at home, begets a
fretfulness at longer confinement. Probably, the dis-
tresses and privations of the family are injudiciously
dwelt upon ; or, some sorrowful tale is told, that
sets the excited brain into such action, that sleep,
which had previously been obtained with great difficulty, is again banished, and the cure consequently
very much retarded. Notwithstanding the know
ledge of these circumstances it is still often very
difficult to know how to decide. It is sometimes
impossible to convince an affectionate husband or
wife, that the sight of one, with whom the patient
has uninterruptedly enjoyed all the endearments of
conjugal life, can possibly be injurious ; and, after
having travelled, perhaps, a distance of thirty or forty
miles, solely for the purpose of seeing a relative, it
is a great disappointment to return without an interview. When interviews are permitted, the friends
should be earnestly cautioned not to dwell upon

painful subjects, but to let the bright side of every thing only be shown. In speaking of this part of the subject, it ought to be mentioned, that interviews with their friends are much less prejudicial when the insanity has arisen from a physical than from a moral cause. In the first instance, the cause cannot be aggravated by it, and if there exists a strong feeling of affection in the parties, it will often soothe and do good; whereas in the latter, these very affections, improperly indulged, are too often the source of the continuation of the disease. It is necessary, therefore, for a much longer time to elapse in these cases before an interview can with safety be permitted, than in the former. But each case must be regulated by its particular circumstances. In many the disease has been much aggravated, and much suffering has been undergone from the neglect, or total forgetfulness of those, upon whose affection they had every claim; but who, having once got rid of the care and charge of them, seem no longer to have retained the slightest anxiety for their welfare. It is at all times desirable, that the person under whose charge the patients are, should hear occasionally from their relatives; so that, on any expression of anxiety for them on the part of the patient, or on any favourable opportunity occurring, to awaken or rouse up a dormant feeling of affection, they may be informed that they are still held in the most affectionate remembrance, and that it is only from prudential motives they have not been permitted to see them.

In asylums exclusively devoted to paupers, it will readily be supposed that many of those admitted are in a state of the grossest ignorance ; and that moral and religious instruction has been too often totally neglected. As the propriety of affording religious instruction to the insane has been often disputed, I think it right to state, that both at Wakefield and at Hanwell the greatest benefit has resulted from it ; and from my experience, I venture to say, it is only when this great moral remedy is indiscriminately and injudiciously applied, that any harm has ever arisen. If a man has had the importance of religious subjects so forcibly impressed upon his mind, that by intense thought upon them he has excited the brain to diseased action, it must be evident, that to attempt to convince him of any error he is at that time labouring under on these subjects, must be injurious, because the very discussion tends to increase the action of those organs, which are already too greatly called into exercise. Under these circumstances, neither religious books nor religious conversation should be permitted ; and the greatest care will be necessary to mark that no excitement on the subject any longer exists, before they are resumed. It is from the nature of insanity not being properly understood, and from the application of even the most useful remedies at improper times, that many of these have fallen into disrepute ; and this has been the case with religious instruction. With few exceptions, the patients, who become deranged on religious subjects, have been persons who have become greatly alarmed on discovering, either from hearing sermons, or reading the word of God, that they have broken his laws, and have been wicked and guilty creatures. Not immediately comprehending the merciful plan of salvation provided for sinners, and therefore not immediately feeling that assurance of pardon and forgiveness which they find is promised in the word of God "to all them that truly repent and unfeignedly believe his holy Gospel," they become greatly distressed, and endeavouring to find out the cause, they fix their attention with the most intense anxiety upon that, to many perplexing and lamentably mistaken passage, " blasphemy against the Holy Ghost ;" and they think, that it is from their having committed this sin they do not derive the same comfort and consolation from religion which thousands possess who believe in the promises of the Gospel. When once this idea has taken hold on the mind, and has been so dwelt upon as to create disordered action in the brain, it is in vain to point out to them, that if they had committed that sin, they would no longer desire to obtain the favour of God; and that their so desiring it is itself a proof they have not committed it; or to point out to them those consoling words of our Saviour, " Him that cometh unto me I will *in no wise* cast out." Neither these nor any other words or arguments can be of use ; medical means must be resorted to, in order to allay the

disordered action of the brain; and the subject of
religion, the moral cause of the insanity, must be
excluded as much as possible from consideration;
and if ever mentioned in conversation with the
patient, of course it should be represented to him
in its most consoling aspect.   A great many confirmed cases of melancholia and suicide take place
from this cause, and very principally from the
premonitory symptoms of the disease being so little
understood.   With the best intentions to do good,
much harm is done by religious conversation and
praying with persons in this state; for though
I by no means intend to say, that if on the coming
on of those perplexing thoughts, the matter can
be put in a light so clear as to satisfy them that
they are not excluded from the favour of God, that
then the anxiety and overaction of the brain would
subside; yet I repeat, that when it has taken place,
every thing of the kind should be avoided.

Though it is acknowledged that much mischief
may arise from injudiciously introducing the subject
of religion in particular cases, I must not omit to mention, that many patients have not only been comforted
by its salutary lessons, whilst they have been in the
asylum, but have retained the benefit after they have
been discharged.   The lessons of instruction have
been carried home to their families; drunkenness
and licentiousness have been forsaken, and temper-
ance, decorum, and piety, substituted in their place.

A. B., a female, about forty-five years of age, a

Roman Catholic, was admitted into the asylum at Wakefield in a state of furious mania brought on from drunkenness. She had lived in one of the large manufacturing towns in the neighbourhood, and kept a brothel; her husband at the same time being a receiver of stolen goods. In addition to this woman's insanity, it was found, after the violence of the paroxysm had abated, that she was as grossly ignorant of all the *vital* truths of Christianity, as she was depraved and abandoned in her conduct. As she began to recover, she was induced, in the first instance, probably as much from curiosity as from any other motive, to attend morning and evening family prayers. Light by degrees broke in upon her mind; she saw the dreadful consequences that would inevitably result from the life she had been leading, and determined, by the help of God, to amend it. She remained in the asylum until she was perfectly restored to sanity, and was so confirmed in the views she had imbibed on religious subjects, that on her return home, she not only gave up all her vicious courses, but had sufficient influence to reform her husband. We had the satisfaction of knowing some years afterwards, that they were continuing to live in respectability, and were members of a Protestant Church.

Neither have the advantages of the religious instruction received in the asylum been confined to persons of grossly immoral and vicious character.

Many, who, although decent in their outward deportment, had, previously to their admission, paid little attention to their religious duties, or had been content with merely going to a place of worship and *saying* prayers, with the form without the power of godliness, have there learnt that all are by nature sinners, and that all, however apparently moral and virtuous, in order to obtain reconciliation and peace with God, to enjoy happiness here in the joyful assurance of happiness hereafter, must humble themselves at the foot of the cross, and seek pardon and remission of sin through the blood of Christ. They have been taught, by the operation of the Spirit upon their hearts, to know from experience the meaning of our Lord's declaration to Nicodemus. They have found the pearl of great price, and they have so estimated its value, that in many instances they have blessed God for having afflicted them, and have esteemed the suffering, painful as it was, which brought them within the sound of the Gospel, and disposed their hearts to receive it, as the happiest event of their lives. They have taken their religion home with them, and have taught it to their children, and they have come back to tell us the joyful news, that to them also the Gospel of Christ has been "the power of God unto salvation."

Before I conclude the observations on the treatment of insanity arising from moral causes, I would add a caution against permitting a patient to have the uncontrolled management of himself too soon after his recovery. For some time after the nervous powers seem to be duly balanced, great care and watchfulness will be required to keep them in that state, especially when the primary cause of the disease is still in existence; and it will frequently be well, after reason seems to be restored, to adopt medical remedies, which the patient would in all probability neglect, if left entirely to himself. It is therefore by far the more prudent course, in these cases, not to allow the patient to return to his home, or to the scenes connected with painful associations, until the weakened brain has had time not only to have recovered its healthy action, but to have acquired vigour and tone. This caution is principally applicable to cases where the insanity has only continued for a comparatively short period. There is a danger of falling into the opposite error when the patient recovers after an attack of some years' continuance. In these instances, when the mind is completely restored, and the patient able to act and judge rationally, there is frequently a very great disinclination to go out again into the world; and, particularly, where much kindness and attention have been experienced during the confinement. The habits become fixed, an attachment is formed to those about them, life is spent without care and anxiety, and a very reasonable fear exists lest the excitement of external objects should induce such an over-action of the brain, as to cause a relapse.

But in these cases it is only right, if the patient continues well for some time, to make the trial, and to restore him to society.

Having considered the treatment of insanity, arising from physical or moral causes, acting primarily on the brain, we will next turn our attention to it when it is produced by the brain sympathizing with some other diseased organ. Many cases of insanity have their origin in diseases of some of the chylopoietic viscera. In all these cases the first object is to restore the secretions to healthy action by the ordinary medical remedies. The same caution, however, which has been previously given, with regard to insanity arising from moral causes, must also be attended to in these cases. The patients will rarely bear excessive bleedings; and it is generally prudent, in the first instance at least, not to use very violent medicines, or to give very large doses. With these exceptions the medical treatment will vary very little from that which would be required if the patient were sane. As the general health is restored the irritation of the brain seems gradually to cease; and, in many cases, the patient recovers, without it being necessary to apply any means for lessening the circulation in the brain. Great attention, however, must always be paid to the state of the head; and, whenever heat or pain in it is found, cold applications and local bleedings should be carefully used. Many patients suffer exceedingly from the insanity being attributed to moral causes when it really arises

from a disease in some of the viscera. Moral remedies are applied whilst the general health is too much
neglected. A striking case of this kind fell under
my observation some years ago. A female, about
forty-five years of age, who went when quite young
into a highly respectable family, as a nursery-maid,
and had continued with them all her life, was observed to be gradually becoming melancholy; and,
from being very active and attentive to her duties,
scarcely to have energy to move about, and to be
so lost in thought as to require rousing before she
could be induced to attend to any thing. The
family became very uneasy about her, the apothecary
usually attending was sent for, and finding the catamenia regular, and being informed that her bowels
were not costive, he considered it a disease of the
mind. This opinion was strengthened by her having
some very gloomy religious views, quite contrary to
her usual disposition. Her affections were apparently altered, and she no longer felt any attachment
to a young man to whom she had long been engaged
to be married. Under these circumstances the attention was given entirely to moral remedies, she was
moved about from place to place, was taken to the
sea coast, and every thing in short was done for her
that could be accomplished by these means. At the
end of five years she was brought, by her kind
master and his amiable daughter, in his carriage to
the asylum, where, after much contention of feeling,
she was left. After making very minute and careful

examination into all the circumstances, I felt persuaded that the cause had been mistaken, and that
instead of the brain being diseased from a cause of
a moral nature acting primarily upon it, it was
affected by sympathy with diseased abdominal viscera.   Acting upon this supposition, a course of
purgatives, alteratives, the warm-bath, and afterwards tonics were persevered in for some time.
The morbid feelings, which from long habit had
become deeply excited, were diverted as much as
possible by employment.   In a few weeks a striking
amendment was visible, and before the expiration of
three months she perfectly recovered, and went back
to her friends.   She afterwards married, and came
to pay us a visit on her wedding excursion.   I do
not recollect having seen any other case so remarkable for the length of time which elapsed before the
proper remedies were applied, in which the patient
recovered : but the proportion of the cures from this
class of patients is by far greater than in those cases
where the insanity arises from physical or moral
causes acting primarily on the brain.

When insanity arises from the suppression of the
natural evacuations, these must of course be relieved,
and in many cases, where it is the result of the sudden stoppage of some artificial discharge, it will be
necessary to re-produce this by medical means.

Insanity, arising from the intemperate use of fermented liquors, is the consequence of the brain
participating in the effects produced on the stomach

through the medium of the nerves; the irritation from the stimulus having been kept up sufficiently long to continue after the absolute stimulus itself has ceased to be supplied. These cases also very generally recover if the diseased action has not been so long continued as to produce diseased structure. It too frequently however happens, that as the "dog returns to his vomit and the sow to her wallowing in the mire," so these patients no sooner feel themselves at liberty, than they begin their old practices : the result is, a speedy return of the insanity; and, if persevered in, paralysis, fatuity, and death. In the young and comparatively healthy class of these patients, on their first attack, little more is necessary than to keep the head cool; diverting the blood to the extremities, and keeping the bowels open, and allaying the irritation by effervescent draughts, combined with small doses of sulphate of magnesia. After the incipient stage is gone off some mild tonic should be administered. When the practice has been long continued, or the patient is in declining years, even if it be a first attack, the collapse is often so great that the patient would sink at once, if all stimulus was immediately to be withheld. A few months ago a person was brought to the asylum at Hanwell, who had formerly been a respectable bookseller, but who from intemperance had sunk in society, until he had become a pauper. He was nearly seventy years of age, and he appeared to be fast sinking into fatuity, and so reduced in bodily health that there was very

little hope of his surviving.   He had only been in
the workhouse a few days, but of course, during that
time, had not been allowed any of his long-continued
potations : his pulse had become intermittent, and
so feeble, it could scarcely be felt, and his appetite
was gone.   In this case, if we had not had recourse
to brandy, the patient would in all probability have
sunk instantly. By the timely application of this stimulus, however, he rallied ; and, by great care, and
with accommodating his diet to his weakened digestive organs, he has got quite well and is discharged.

Cases of Puerperal Insanity, prior to delivery, are
not very numerous in public hospitals.   Sympathy
with the uterus and with the morbid action of the
stomach and bowels is generally the cause.   Unless
there is a strong hereditary tendency to the disease,
or the patient is of a peculiarly nervous temperament,
an attack of this kind seldom supervenes, when the
secretions from all these organs proceed in the natural way ; at the same time there is no doubt, but that
the various circumstances of hope and fear in which
females are necessarily placed at such times, render
them more sensitive than usual to the operations of
a variety of moral impressions. It has been known
to come on at every period of gestation : it is usually
accompanied by some inflammatory diathesis, and
antiphlogistic remedies and bleeding should be applied ; great caution should be observed in the use of
them, particularly of the latter.   The cases I have
seen very generally improved as the time of gestation

drew nigh, and all entirely recovered a few weeks
after delivery.   Very few of the cases of puerperal
insanity, after delivery, are brought to the asylum
at Hanwell, until after the lapse of many weeks or
months.   The lacteal and other secretions are generally in diseased action, if not entirely suppressed.
The first thing to be attended to is to restore these
to a healthy state: the warm-bath, diaphoretics, gentle
aperients, camphor mixture combined with tincture
digitalis, or tincture hyoscyami, are often very useful
in procuring sleep ; but the shaving of the head and
the persevering in applications of cold are the best
means of lessening the irritability in this, as in every
stage of acute insanity.   If the treatment be commenced in the early stage of the disease, and there
is no hereditary predisposition or powerful moral
cause to keep up diseased action in the brain, it is
one of the most curable forms of insanity.   Puerperal
insanity sometimes arises from excessive hemorrhage.   This may take place at any period of gestation after the third or fourth month, but it most
frequently happens immediately on delivery : the
brain becomes incapable of performing its functions
aright, from not receiving a due supply of blood.   In
these cases the powers of the constitution must be
restored by tonics, and a mild nutritious diet given
frequently, but in small quantities : moderate exercise in the open air should be used, the bowels should
be kept tolerably open, and all excitement, particularly the presence and conversation of relations and

friends, should, as much as possible, be avoided. The mental faculties are usually found to improve with the general health and strength of the patient. During the whole time that puerperal insanity exists, and more especially during the first periods of it, the strictest watchfulness is requisite to prevent the patient from committing suicide; for there is no form of insanity in which attempts at self-destruction are more unexpectedly and suddenly made than in this. It very usually happens, that the most perfect indifference is shown by the mother to her child; indeed it is neither safe nor proper to allow it to come to her until some favourable change has taken place : but as soon as it can be done with safety, and the affections excited by it, a new train of feelings is at once called into action, and this has the most beneficial tendency.

We will now consider the treatment of cases of insanity, where the brain, from any cause, does not appear to receive an adequate supply of blood. It has been already stated, that in inanition, want of an adequate supply of food has been in many cases the apparent cause of the disease, although even in these instances it may be difficult to exclude, as an exciting cause, the operation of anxiety, which necessarily accompanies great distress of circumstances. In these cases there is great languor, and a feeble pulse; the bowels are torpid, and the patient generally suffers from the long catalogue of dyspeptic symptoms. The bodily health must be restored, and a mild, nutritious, but by no means stimulating, diet must be administered. The head must be kept cool ; and as the strength will permit, if it is exceedingly hot, or there is much pain in it, small local bleedings may be used with advantage. We have already noticed the mode of treatment where the brain is deprived of its due supply of blood from hemorrhages attending gestation. Pro-- fuse hemorrhages, from any other cause, will, in like manner, produce insanity, and the treatment of it must be similar.

The only remaining cases of incipient insanity, which it will be necessary to notice, are those caused by the pernicious practice previously alluded to. The medical reader is referred to the note at the end of the volume, corresponding to the page.

We will next proceed to the treatment of cases of insanity where the disease has become chronic. When we consider the little information generally possessed as to the nature of the disease, the neglect in making timely application, and the improper treatment in the early stages, we shall not be surprised that a very great number remain for life uncured. In large pauper establishments, particularly on their being first opened, the greater part of the patients admitted consists of those who have been long under confinement, and who are consigned to them as their permanent abode. Indeed, the fact that the lunatics belonging to the counties are not placed in circumstances favourable for their cure, is the very reason why county asylums are built; and unless they are sufficiently large to hold the paupers, insane at the time of their being opened, and also to admit those, who are subsequently attacked, as soon as the disease makes its appearance, they become entirely filled with old cases; and before the recent ones can possibly be taken in, weeks or months must elapse, and the opportunity of cure is lost. This has been particularly the case with the asylum at Hanwell. At the time when it was contemplated, it was known that there were upwards of eight hundred lunatics chargeable to the county of Middlesex, and to the different parishes in it, in confinement. It was originally built to hold three hundred patients, but was soon filled almost entirely with old cases. As no patients can be discharged except on their being cured, or on the undertaking of their friends to provide for them, that is, on their ceasing to be paupers, the only other vacancies arise from deaths; and as the exercise, the pure air, and wholesome diet at Hanwell, greatly tend to prolong life, the mortality has been very small: indeed, the epileptic and consumptive have formed a great proportion of the deaths in each year. From these circumstances it has, with scarcely any exception, been impossible to admit the recent cases on their first becoming insane; and before they can be taken in, the most favourable opportunity for the application of medical and moral remedies has passed away. Indeed, as the parishes claim the right to send a number of paupers, in proportion to their rental, it frequently happens that when application is made by a parish for the admission of a recent case, the parish has its full number in the asylum ; and that when a vacancy does occur, it must be filled up, not by the recent case, but by an old and incurable patient from another parish, that has a right to the vacancy. When alterations were made in the asylum, and it was rendered able to contain rather more than double the number for which it was originally built ; yet as the additional accommodation was not sufficient to hold one half of those who were then confined in the different private asylums and workhouses, of course the class of patients admitted, still continued to be the old and incurable. But much may be done even for these : the severity of the exacerbation may be abated, and the time of its duration shortened, and the patients may enjoy a considerable share of comfort and happiness between the attacks.

We have already stated, that we believe that insanity arises in the first instance from diseased action of the brain and nervous system, and that if this diseased action remains unchecked, diseased organization of the brain or its membranes, to a greater or less extent, follows. Whenever any portion of the brain or its membranes has become thus permanently injured, its functions can never again be perfectly performed ; and we have a complete case of chronic insanity. In some cases the

lesion is comparatively trifling, and the derangement is confined to matters so unimportant in the
common duties of life, that though it cannot be said
that no injurious alteration in the character has
taken place, yet so many faculties are still left
unimpaired, that the patient is capable of managing
his affairs; and unless something occurs to excite
the diseased part to excessive action, no symptom
of derangement may be exhibited for weeks or even
months together.   In fact, from the organs of the
brain being double, a portion of one hemisphere may
be diseased, and even to a considerable extent; and
still, in the absence of excitement, the ordinary operations may be performed in such a way as not to call
forth particular observation.   But whenever diseased
organization really exists, however small its extent,
there is a great liability to positive attacks of insanity:
and each succeeding attack tends still further to
add to the diseased organization, and to weaken the
mental powers. In some cases these attacks recur at
regular periods; in others, the intervals of convalescence vary, and seem to depend upon the continued absence of any exciting cause, physical or
moral. In many, where the lesion has proceeded to
a great extent, and the patient at all times exhibits
decided symptoms of derangement, there is a similar
liability to exacerbations ; and a very slight exciting
cause, physical or moral, is often sufficient to bring
them on.   I have known several cases, where they
have been produced merely from the nervous excite-

ment arising from a slight cold, or even from the
toothache. Many patients, who suffer extremely from
them, and who are in consequence very much reduced, and made very thin, remain well until they
attain a certain degree of plumpness : as soon as this
appears, another attack may be expected.   In these
cases, of course, great care must be used in regulating
the patients' diet ; as they may, by proper management, frequently escape an attack for many months.
In the intervals of the attacks, many of the functions
are performed so well, that although the patient is
not at any time capable of managing his own affairs,
he may be usefully and happily employed.   The
symptoms of the attacks, in the chronic cases, are
very similar to those already mentioned, as preceding and accompanying incipient insanity : the head
becomes hot, the secretions are disordered, the patient is irritable, and there is an alteration for the
worse in his general manner and conduct.   As soon
as any of these symptoms are observed, the system
previously pointed out, as proper to be adopted on
the commencement of insanity, should be at once
pursued, but with a still greater caution in the use of
depleting remedies.   By carefully watching the first
appearance of these symptoms, and at once keeping
the patient perfectly quiet, and applying the small
local bleedings and other medical remedies, the attack, which, if the patient were not properly attended
to, would last for many weeks, may be frequently
stopped in the course of a few days, and with

comparatively but little increased diseased organization of the brain. I can speak with some degree
of confidence, as to the effect of local bleedings in
chronic cases. Many patients have been under my
care who afford an opportunity of forming a correct
estimate of its effect. Under the old system, the
exacerbations were severe and of long continuance;
and, although it is universally acknowledged, that
the longer the patient remains insane, the more difficult and tedious is each succeeding attack to be
cured, I have no hesitation in saying, that by the
adoption of the local bleedings, and of the plan previously pointed out, the violence of the attacks has
been diminished, and their duration shortened. In
fact, where the patient used to suffer for months,
under the ordinary course of merely attending to the
secretions, and keeping him as free as possible from
excitement, he is now frequently restored in a few
days, by the application of this system, on the very
first appearance of an approaching attack. In the
intervals of the attacks, employment, according to
the various capacities of the patients, combined with
firm and kind moral treatment, on the plan previously mentioned, is the best means of increasing
their general health, of contributing to their comfort, and of prolonging the period of their convalescence. In many cases, where the disease has been of
long standing, and the mind has become habituated to
an erroneous train of thinking, a careful perseverance
in this plan has gradually prolonged the periods

of comparative convalescence, and diminished the length and violence of the exacerbations, until the attention has become occupied, and the mind by degrees been weaned from its morbid feelings; and the patient has eventually become sane, and been restored to society. Of course, in these cases, a very great susceptibility of disease remains; and any excitement, particularly immediately on recovery, will most probably produce a relapse. Unfortunately, when a poor man, who has been for a long time an inmate of a lunatic asylum, where his daily wants have been supplied without any care or anxiety on his part, becomes sane, there is great difficulty in introducing him again into the world, and making him entirely dependent upon his own exertions, without at the same time producing a greater feeling of anxiety than his enfeebled brain and nervous system are capable of bearing. Many of the paupers, on their recovery, are entirely without resources; and they are driven of necessity into the workhouses, until they can obtain employment: this is more than they are able to bear. The benevolence of a gentleman of the name of Harrison, has done much to relieve cases of this kind, occurring in the West Riding of Yorkshire. Her Majesty Queen Adelaide is the patroness of a charity, which has for its object the supply of the immediate and most pressing necessities of the paupers, when discharged cured, from the asylum at Hanwell. Her Majesty contributed to it one hundred pounds, and other sums have already been subscribed, which have raised the amount of Queen Adelaide's Fund to the sum of nearly one thousand eight hundred pounds : this has been invested in the funds ; and the dividends have, in several instances, been the means of affording such timely assistance, as has, in all probability, prevented a relapse, and enabled the convalescent to maintain himself in comfort and respectability.   But something further is still wanted. A comfortable place, where such of the patients as might be deemed proper objects, might, for a time, find food and shelter, and a home, until they could procure employment, would be an invaluable blessing to them ; and if such an institution were established, even at the cost of the parishes, it would in the end prove a saving.   Many patients might be tried in such an establishment, and eventually restored to society, who are now compelled to remain in the asylum as lunatics, in consequence of their retaining some erroneous view, on some unimportant matter.   Although this does not interfere with their capability of judging between right and wrong, or prevent them from performing their duty, it is an insurmountable bar to a medical superintendent signing a certificate of their sanity ; and, without this, the visiting justices cannot order their discharge.   I have no doubt, that in many instances, this erroneous impression would be effaced by a little mixing in the world, and in the ordinary business of life : indeed I have known cases of this kind, where the friends have made the trial, and have procured the discharges of the patients, on the undertaking, that they shall be no longer a burden to the parish. The greatest success has been the result : the complete change of scene, and the occupation of mind have entirely diverted the thoughts from the subject, on which the erroneous impression remained; and as this ceased to be dwelt upon, the derangement gradually wore off, and the patient soon became perfectly sane. The friends of several of the patients would gladly venture to make the experiment for a few weeks, but they are afraid of undertaking the maintenance of them permanently. This difficulty might be obviated by providing such a retreat as has just been mentioned : but even if this be impracticable, much might be done by permitting the patients when convalescent, at proper times, to go out and mix with the world before their discharge. Unfortunately, so strong a feeling against this plan exists in the county of Middlesex, that its adoption at the asylum at Hanwell is, for the present at least, quite out of the question. In old cases, amongst the affluent, where no pressing anxiety exists for the supply of the daily wants, there can be no doubt but that a change of residence, and even a return into the domestic circle, ought to be much more frequently tried than is usually the case. After a time the violence of the disease subsides, but the monotony which exists in the small situations, in which they are usually confined, offers nothing to divert the mind. Erroneous impressions become rooted, and although these are frequently limited to matters of trifling importance, they are sufficient to prevent the patient from being certified to be perfectly sane, or, at all events, they justify his being detained. Without some change of scene there is but little hope of improvement. In many of these cases an introduction again into the world, or into the domestic circle, would complete the restoration, and the trial might be made without risk.

I cannot conclude this chapter without adding a few observations on a subject which materially affects the treatment of the insane ; I mean, the medical education of those under whose care they are placed. It is perfectly inconsistent with common sense to suppose that a man shall intuitively know how to treat insanity. We have seen, that although in the greater number of cases it is attended with the same general result, yet it assumes most varied forms, and great care and discrimination are required in the treatment : indeed, it is universally acknowledged to be a most difficult and mysterious disease, and yet it is almost the only one on which the medical student receives no particular instruction. In his attendance on the hospitals he will, in all probability, have met with almost every other variety of disease which afflicts human nature ; at all events, his lectures will have supplied him with some information as to their treatment : but I believe that my friend and colleague, Dr. Morison of Cavendish Square, is the only lecturer in London, expressly on insanity ; and I understand that he has not a large class. Indeed, except as being incidentally touched upon in the lectures on forensic medicine, it appears almost entirely neglected in the course of a medical education ; and, as the subject does not form a branch of examination, the pupils naturally employ their time in those studies which will be directly available, and assist them in the obtaining their medical certificates : the result is, that professional men, in other respects well educated, commence practice almost in a state of total ignorance on the subject. This is an evil from which every individual, whatever be his rank or fortune, is liable to suffer in his own person, and in that of his friends : and a man of ingenuous mind can hardly be placed under more painful circumstances, than to find the father or mother of a family, in a state of insanity, entrusted to his care, and to feel conscious that upon him depends the restoration of the patient to reason and happiness, whilst his want of acquaintance with the disease renders him unfit for the task, and he knows not where to apply for advice. This is by no means an imaginary evil, it is one of frequent occurrence ; and numerous are the instances, where amiable and valuable members of society are consigned for life to a perpetual banishment from their friends, in the gloom of a madhouse, solely from ignorance on the part of the medical adviser. This ought to be remedied :—the first step would be, not to permit any student to be qualified to pass an examination, either as a physician, surgeon, or apothecary, without producing certificates of having previously attended course of lectures on insanity ; and it ought to form as usual a subject of examination as any other disease. There would be considerable difficulties at the first, especially in obtaining teachers properly qualified, in the provincial schools; but in this, as in other things, the demand will create the supply.   When the time and labour required for the acquisition of knowledge of the subject receive an adequate remuneration, men of the greatest ability in the profession will devote their attention to it; and the investigation which it will receive from those who are about to deliver lectures upon it will, eventually, throw much light upon the disease.   In connexion with insanity I should strongly recommend the study of phrenology: the tendency which it gives carefully to note, and the facility with which it enables us easily to distinguish variations in conduct, which, though minute, and apparently of little consequence, are, in reality, the marks of important changes of action in the brain, would alone be sufficient to recommend it to our most serious attention.   But I have no hesitation in saying, that in addition to its being indirectly useful, in thus helping us to a more accurate acquaintance with the state of the patient, it may be applied directly to most valuable purposes.   One instance of its use has already been detailed : I could mention others, where the mere examination of the head, without any previous knowledge or information whatever as to the habits of the patient, has suggested the trial of a particular course of moral treatment, which subsequent events have fully proved to be correct.   Nor will this be a matter of surprise, when we remember that those organs, through the action of which the grand distinctions of character are produced, form large masses of brain, and that to distinguish their relative size and natural operation, it is not necessary to have recourse to callipers, or to determine their extent to a hair's breadth. A single glance will show, to a person in the habit of observing, whether the formation of the head indicates a naturally bold and passionate, or a timid and retiring man; will enable us to distinguish between one highly gifted with the intellectual and nobler faculties, and consequently proportionally responsible for their active and continued employment, with direct reference to the glory of God, and his neighbour, less liberally endowed, who has to struggle against a constitutional tendency towards mere animal gratification,—a struggle of a different kind, but not more difficult to be overcome, than the natural disposition to divert the higher powers of the mind from their true end, and to devote them to the contemplation and service of the creature instead of the Creator.

I am aware that the instruction obtained from the mere attendance upon lectures would not be sufficient to qualify a professional man for undertaking the moral as well as the medical management; but the knowledge that would, by this means, be gained of the premonitory symptoms, would frequently prevent an attack of insanity coming on : at all events it would relieve the patient from the danger of being exposed to permanent loss of reason from injudicious treatment, on its commencement. Clinical lectures have been very strongly recommended; and, if the instruction of the pupils were the only object, there can be no doubt that they ought to be adopted : but it must be remembered, that the first things to be considered are the cure and welfare of the patients; and, any one *practically* conversant with the disease will, I am sure, acknowledge, that the excitement which would be produced in the minds of the patients by a number of pupils going round an asylum, in the same manner as they go round an hospital, would be most prejudicial; in many cases it would entirely prevent recovery. This, therefore, as a general practice, can never be adopted; but there would be no objection to permit such members of the profession, as determined to apply themselves exclusively or more particularly to the study of this disease, to attend public asylums daily. They might be valuable auxiliaries in the institution : they would become acquainted with the details of its management, and conversant with every varied form of the disease, and the treatment, both moral and medical, which ought to be adopted. They would be fitted either to take the management of public institutions, or, in addition to their private practice, to deliver lectures, and to impart useful and valuable knowledge to others. But, in order that the insane may really be placed under the most favourable circumstances, the instruction ought not to be confined to our sex. Strong

prejudices, and very improper feelings, have long
existed against females in any degree above the class
of servants, being employed so as to obtain a liveli-
hood for themselves, except as governesses. Any
other occupation has been considered as degrading.
But I hope a brighter day is dawning upon society,
and that the application by females of the higher
classes of their abilities to useful purposes, will soon
cease to be a matter of surprise. There can be little
doubt of the effect of such a change upon their own
happiness. They would be cheerful and contented,
they would escape ennui, and would no longer have
occasion to avail themselves of the thousand contrivances, to which the idle are obliged to resort, to get
rid of time : and the result of such an addition of
useful labour would be a great increase to the happiness of mankind. I know no way in which female
kindness and ability could be more beneficially employed, than in obtaining the requisite information,
and then taking charge of the insane. A wife, a
sister, or a daughter exhibits an alteration in manner, which indicates the existence of diseased action
in the brain—there is a morbid sensitiveness of feeling—it is essential that she should at once be taken
from her home, and be entrusted to strangers. Can
any one doubt the advantage of securing as her com-
panion, a lady of tender feelings, of refined and cultivated mind, and who has had such a portion of
nstruction on the disease, as to enable her carefully
and judiciously to apply, under the direction of the

professional man, proper medical and moral treatment? Is there a husband, a father, or a brother who would not hail as a benefactress, a female so endowed and so instructed, who would take the charge of his relative? If such be the obvious utility of a well-informed and judicious lady to take the charge of a single patient, it is unnecessary to point out the importance of those who are the matrons of public asylums, being properly educated for the purpose. I do not mean that females should attend a dissecting-room, or enter upon a course of the study of medicine, but it would be most desirable that they should have an opportunity of obtaining a sound and fundamental knowledge of the various modes in which diseased action of the brain exhibits itself in the conduct, and of the dangers to be guarded against, and of the moral treatment which ought to be adopted.

CHAPTER VII.

ON APOPLEXY, EPILEPSY, AND THE DISEASES OF THE INSANE.

I STATED, in the early part of this work, that I rather consider apoplexy to be a variety of that disease of the brain and nervous system, which produces insanity in one person, epilepsy in another, and convulsions in a third, than a frequent, direct cause of insanity itself. Apoplectic attacks alone, however, when purely sanguineous, are undeniably often followed by insanity. This arises from the injury the brain has sustained either from fulness in the vessels, or, more likely, from some extravasation on a part capable of bearing it without fatal consequences; though death is generally the immediate result in the latter case. The insanity which follows apoplexy is usually attended with some degree of paralysis, especially in the organs of speech. Sometimes only a very little stammering is observed, but this by degrees increases until the nerves, both of motion and feeling, lose their action. The prognosis in all these cases is unfavourable : the patient very soon sinks under extensive sloughings. The integuments in every part, especially in the extremities, lose their vitality to such a degree, that the mere pressure of one part of the body against another is sufficient to destroy its structure.

I do not pretend to understand how these things are, nor can I suggest a remedy; but it is to be hoped, from the diligent researches into the nervous system now making by Sir C. Bell, Dr. Marshall Hall, and other intelligent gentlemen, that more light will soon be thrown upon it.

One of the most distressing, because one of the most incurable forms of insanity, is that in which it is combined with epilepsy. I am totally at a loss to explain how it is that we find morbid structure of the bones, hydatids, pus, and other extraneous substances in the brain, producing in one patient a continued state of insanity; in another epilepsy, recurring at regular periods, and attended with no defect of intellect after the convulsions cease; in another, epilepsy, followed by the most furious mania for many successive days, even after the fits have ceased altogether; but these varieties in the disease are well known. *Post-mortem* examination usually discovers much cerebral disease, several ounces of serum are also found in the ventricles, and under the membranes. In all large establishments the epileptic form a considerable portion of the inmates: in the asylum at Hanwell, sixty-three out of six hundred and eight are affected with it. I have myself tried, and seen my medical colleagues try, all the usual remedies, such as setons, blisters, vomits, purges, bleedings, sedatives, mercury, and numerous other things, likely and unlikely; but I do not recollect ever seeing any benefit arise from the use of them, when the seat of disease appeared in the head, and accompanied insanity. In most cases, both the frequency and the violence of the fits may be prevented by strict attention to diet, keeping the bowels open, and avoiding all sources of mental irritation. In the instance of a female about eighteen years of age, where the cause of irritation appeared to be in the intestines, turpentine was of great use; and she perfectly recovered after taking it for some time. But it is well known, that whenever epilepsy arises from the irritation of teething, worms, or other diseases in the stomach and intestines, the removal of the cause will very probably cure the disease.

The insane are of course liable to accidents and illness, in common with the rest of mankind; but with the exception of their being constantly subject to diseases peculiarly connected with the nervous system, and which, notwithstanding what has been said to the contrary, I am decidedly of opinion tend to shorten life, they are not, when under proper management, a sickly class. It is probable that this may, in a great measure, arise from the regularity of their diet, habits, &c. Another reason may be, that cold, damp, and other circumstances which, in the sane, bring on sore throats, inflammation of the lungs, or other complaints, according to the particular idiosyncrasies, frequently produce in the insane diseased action of the brain : but, independently of diseases peculiarly connected with the nervous system, the insane seem particularly subject to others, such as chronic inflammation of the mucous membrane of the bowels, diarrhœa, and dysentery. These diseases appear to depend a good deal on locality : in the Asylum at Wakefield, a large proportion of the deaths was at one time owing to them; whilst, in the one at Hanwell, they are comparatively of rare occurrence ; this probably may be accounted for, by the former being on a cold clay soil, and the latter on a fine bed of dry gravel. Consumption, too, is a very frequent cause of the termination of their existence; and very large and numerous tubercles are often seen on dissection, when no expectoration of pus whatever had previously taken place. As the treatment of any disease by which the insane are attacked is the same as that pursued with the sane, it is unnecessary to say more on the subject : it should, however, always be borne in mind, that as the nervous system in general is under diseased action, all the remedies applied should be used with caution, and this ought to be particularly attended to in the use of depletions, and in the exhibition of vegetable poisons.

CHAPTER VIII.

ON THE CONSTRUCTION OF ASYLUMS, AND THE MODE OF THEIR MANAGEMENT.

It has been already stated, as essential to the cure of the disease, that some place should be provided for the insane, where they can be kept separate from their relatives, and those persons whom they have been in the habit of commanding; and where they will be removed from all objects likely to re-produce the same train of thinking which accompanied, if it did not bring on, the attack. For the poor, no place can be found which will bear any comparison with a County Lunatic Asylum: their wants are there provided for in the most substantial manner, and at an expense which is but little felt by each individual who contributes to it: and, as no one in such establishments has the least advantage by the patients remaining in them, they are sure to be discharged as soon as they are sufficiently recovered to justify such a step. Wherever there are one hundred lunatic paupers in one county, there ought to be an asylum; or, if two small counties, adjoining each other, can agree to build one according to the provisions of the 9 Geo. IV., it would be still more advantageous, as the expense of providing for them

necessarily decreases in the ratio of the number in
the institution.   Having determined upon the building, the next consideration is the site. It is of great
importance that it should be elevated, and by no
means in a cold or exposed situation : the soil ought,
if possible, to be gravel or chalk.   It is absolutely
essential that there should be such an abundance of
water, that it should be perfectly immaterial whether
a thousand gallons, or a thousand hogsheads, a day
are used. In addition to any supply of spring water
that may be furnished, I strongly recommend, that
all the rain water should be collected from the roof,
in a separate tank ; it will be at all times valuable for
washing, brewing, or other domestic purposes. The
building should be at such a distance from any town
that a very considerable portion of land around it
may be purchased at a cheap rate.   The quality of
the ground, if it be improvable, is not of so much
consequence as the quantity ; the manual labour of
the patients, in a few years, rendering almost any
ground productive, if the soil and manure from the
establishment be properly secured. With respect to
the form of the building, I rather prefer three sides
of a rectangular parallelogram to any other, with the
centre about double the length of the sides.   The
residence of the superintendent and matron, with
the various business offices, should be placed in the
middle of the centre ; and behind these should be
the kitchens, sculleries, washhouse, bakehouse, brew-
house, &c. &c., so as to admit of easy access from the
centre. The wards for the males should occupy one

side, those for the females, the other side of the
building. If the whole of the ground-floor is elevated, which it ought to be, in order that it may be
perfectly dry at all seasons, a passage may very easily
be made in the basement, from the kitchen to the
extreme corners of the central part of the building,
along which the provisions, &c. &c. may be conveyed
from the various domestic offices, and from these
corners, to the different wards of both the male and
female patients. The gardens, farm-yard, and all
other buildings connected with the out-door labour,
should be placed at the back of the various offices,
from which there should be easy access to them.
The airing courts for the wards, in the centre of the
building, will be on each side of the domestic offices, and, of course, completely separated from each
other ; those for the side-wings ought to be placed
on the east and west sides. If it can be conveniently
managed, the entrance to the building should be on
the north side, as it is much more cheerful to have
the galleries in which the patients walk to front the
south ; and it is never well for them to be so placed
as to be able to see all the persons coming and going
to the asylum. Having thus given a general outline
of the building, let us now proceed to enter a little
more into detail. I am afraid that this will be dry
and uninteresting ; although, from my having been
continually in the habit of receiving letters from
persons concerned in the erection of asylums, both
at home and abroad, requesting an opinion on the
minutiæ, I hope it will not be altogether useless.

The arrangements here mentioned are by no means thought incapable of improvement; but they are selected after visiting and seeing the plans of a great number of lunatic asylums, both at home and on the continent, and after twenty years' residence in two of the largest in England.

The first object that should be kept in view, after providing for the comfort and health of the patients, is economy: for, after all that can be said of the feelings of humanity towards this unfortunate class of our fellow-creatures, their sufferings are too much out of sight to create that sympathy for them which is felt for others, whose wants are more known. It becomes necessary then to show, that to render them efficient assistance need cost very little more than to neglect them: indeed, if the probability of cure be taken into consideration, it is in reality to the pecuniary advantage of each county to provide asylums sufficiently large to hold *all* their lunatics.

But whilst we keep economy in view, we must take care that we are not misled in supposing that things procured for the least money are always the cheapest. In purchasing the site of ground for the building of the asylum at Hanwell, a high price was given for it, in comparison with that for which land could have been bought at Fryarn Barnet, the only other place in which any was offered at all likely to answer the purpose; but yet, from its proximity to the Grand Junction Canal, which will be observed by referring to the Plan at the beginning of this work, all the materials wanted for the erection of the building were brought by water.   It will, therefore, be easily comprehended, that the ground selected for the site was by far the cheaper place of the two ; indeed, I am informed by Mr. Sibley, who was the county surveyor at that time, that the difference of cost to the county, in having the materials by that conveyance, instead of the mode by which they must have been conveyed to Fryarn Barnet, amounted to more than the fee simple of the land.   The permanent advantage, too, of receiving by canal all the heavy materials in daily use, in so large an establishment, is found to be a great saving : in the coals alone, the difference of the expense between the carriage of the quantity consumed, to Hanwell, instead of to Fryarn Barnet, is nearly equal to the interest of the money expended in the purchase of the land.

But in the choice of a site for the building, one consideration ought to weigh more even than economy, that is health.   The advantage of having a healthy situation for establishments of this kind, is of the utmost importance ; and the benefit of it has been felt, in a peculiar manner, at Hanwell.   Notwithstanding few patients are received there until organic disease of the brain has taken place, to such an extent that they are incurable when admitted, yet the air is so salubrious, that the deaths, in proportion to the average number of patients in the house, are fewer than in any other large pauper establishment in the kingdom, where all who come in remain until they die, or are discharged cured, or cease to be paupers.

The following is a list, for the last six years, of the average number of patients at Lancaster, Wakefield, and Hanwell, the largest asylums in the kingdom, and of the corresponding deaths. These annual averages could not be taken from an earlier period, as the asylum at Hanwell was not opened for the reception of patients until the 15th of May, 1831. The salubrity of the air at Hanwell seems to avert much of the virulence of epidemics. During the period in which the patients laboured under the Cholera, the mortality from that awful disease was comparatively small; and, although the Influenza prevailed for some time, only one or two patients died in consequence of it.

Average number of Patients and number of their deaths in the following years, at the County Lunatic Asylum at Lancaster.

Year ending 23 March.	Average number of Patients.	Deaths.			
		Males.	Females.	Total.	Per Cent.
1832	$343\frac{125}{365}$	42	27	69	20.09
1833	$313\frac{100}{365}$	87	60	*147	46.92
1834	$319\frac{308}{365}$	41	24	65	20.32
1835	$360\frac{66}{365}$	30	25	55	15.27
1836	$400\frac{252}{365}$	40	36	76	18.96
1837	$411\frac{149}{365}$	56	54	†110	26.73
	$2148\frac{270}{365} = 2148.7$ nearly			522	

And 2148.7 : 100 :: 522 : 24.29.

Average annual per centage of deaths during the last six years, 24.29.

---

* Of whom 94 died from Cholera.

† Of whom 46 died from Phthisis *after* Influenza.

Average number of Patients, and number of their Deaths in the following years, at the County Lunatic Asylum, at Wakefield.

Year ending 31 Dec.	Average number of Patients.	Deaths.			
		Males.	Females.	Total.	Per Cent.
1832	286	35	18	53	18.53
1833	302	31	21	52	17.21
1834	303	22	21	43	14.19
1835	303	30	30	60	19.80
1836	309	32	24	56	18.12
1837	321	34	28	62	19.31
	1824			326	

And 1824 : 100 :: 326 : 17.87.

Average annual per centage of deaths during the last six years, 17.87.

Average number of Patients, and the number of their Deaths in the following years, at the County Lunatic Asylum at Hanwell.

Year ending 31 Dec.	Average number of Patients.	Deaths.			
		Males.	Females.	Total.	Per Cent.
1832	427	46	53	*99	23.18
1833	537	46	31	77	14.33
1834	564	35	23	58	10.28
1835	580	45	26	71	12.24
1836	611	43	22	65	10.63
1837	608	24	24	48	7.89
	3327			418	

And 3327 : 100 :: 418 : 12.56.

Average annual per centage of deaths during the last six years, 12.56.

---

* Of whom 11 died from Cholera.

It will be seen from these tables, that taking the average per centage of deaths, for the last six years, it is, at

Lancaster	24.29	⎰ and taking the relative pro-	⎱	4
Wakefield,	17.87	⎰ portion in round numbers,	⎱	3
Hanwell,	12.56	⎱ it differs very little from	⎰	2

From the professional skill and zeal of the medical gentlemen at Lancaster and Wakefield, this difference in the mortality can only be accounted for from the singularly healthy situation of the asylum at Hanwell.

The building should be as plain as possible; at the same time, a plan displaying taste, with an imposing appearance, at no more cost than one without these qualifications, ought certainly to be preferred. The first entering into the confines of such establishments often produces a salutary effect upon the mind of a patient, if the aspect is agreeable, and the contrary when otherwise. The building itself ought to be of brick or stone, and in every part fire-proof: the roof should be of iron; indeed an iron roof can now be procured at as cheap a rate as a wooden one of the same strength. In the roof should be placed cisterns for hot and cold water, which ought to be distributed by pipes to all the wards and offices.

An important saving may be effected by having the building three stories high. I am aware that great objections have been made to this arrangement, particularly in France; but I think, without sufficient reason: the epileptic, and those likely to injure themselves in going down stairs, may be placed on the ground-floor. Any objection to the plan from its fancied inconvenience to the servants is perfectly futile ; there are, and very properly, so many contrivances to prevent the necessity of their leaving their wards, that their journeys up and down stairs are much less frequent than those of servants in private families. This plan was found to answer exceedingly well in the asylum at Wakefield, where I resided for many years ; and, as it effects a considerable saving, I have no hesitation in recommending it. One keeper ought not to have under his charge more than twenty, or twenty-five, patients at the most ; and it is more convenient for each ward to contain that number only, than for them to be larger, with two keepers to each. There ought to be a dining room for every fifty patients. When the building is sufficiently large to admit of two wards, each containing from twenty to twenty-five patients on the same floor, in each of the side wings, and of two male and of two female wards, of similar size, in the centre, there should be a dining room on each floor, in the centre of each side wing, for the two side wards ; and one on each floor, between the two male wards, in the centre of the building, and a similar one between the two female wards. These rooms can also be used for the patients to work in ; and from this position the keepers can easily inspect the patients whilst walking in the galleries. In a building of this magnitude, two of the adjoining wards on each side of the house ought to be thrown into one, for the purpose of being converted into a walk for spinning string. This occupation is, indeed, so conducive to the comfort of the patients, that where the size of the building will not admit of such a spinning walk being in the galleries, a covered way ought to be erected for the express purpose. Where each wing contains only one ward on a floor, having twenty-five patients in each, the dining room for the fifty patients ought to be at the corner, and should be so constructed as to give easy inspection into the side, and also into the centre ward. The tables in the dining rooms should be fixed in such a manner, that the patients can sit at their seats, fastened into the walls of the room : they need not be wide, as it is convenient for one side not to be occupied by the patients. There ought to be a proportion of about sixty-six separate sleeping apartments for every hundred patients. The sleeping apartments, for single patients, should not be less than eight feet six inches long, and six feet nine inches wide, and twelve feet high. At Hanwell each sleeping apartment contains six hundred and sixty cubic feet. As a general principle, I should prefer having the sleeping apartments only on one side of the gallery ; but in a county asylum for paupers, there will always be a considerable portion in so helpless a state of fatuity, as to be unable to appreciate any of the advantages of a cheerful aspect ; and, if they have a pure air to breathe, are kept clean, kindly attended to, and well fed, nothing more can be done for them. For this class of patients, the more economical plan of having the sleeping apartments on each side of the galleries may be adopted with propriety : to obviate however, the darkness, and to give even these galleries a degree of cheerfulness, open spaces, sufficiently large to contain beds, may be left on each side of the gallery; in which windows should be placed for light and air. The patients may dine as well as sleep in these spaces, the bedding being removed, during the day, to an adjoining apartment : this arrangement will save the expense of a separate dining room for patients of this class. Each ward ought to contain a small warm bath, and also a sink and a water-closet. Though the matter may appear trifling, the alteration of these, if not made on a good plan at the first, is afterwards a source of considerable annoyance and expense : the sinks have usually a trap, made immediately on the pipe descending from the stone; and, as the trap is seldom more than one inch deep, it very soon becomes choked up; and it must, therefore, be continually taken up, which is very troublesome; or it must be left loose, in which case we find, that the patients cram various articles down the pipe, and in this mode prevent the water running off. The best plan to obviate this nuisance, is to have a proper grating fixed upon the mouth of the pipe, with a trap a little lower down, made in the shape of the letter S. Any thing that will pass through the grating can then easily go through the rest of the pipe. With respect to the water-closets, unless great care is used, both by the architect in forming them, and by the keepers afterwards, in watching the patients, it will cost a considerable sum to keep them in order ; and they will be frequently choked up, and create a great nuisance. A long trough, placed at a convenient inclination under the seat, with a grate about one foot from that end of it which communicates with the descending pipe, seems to answer very well. Over the part between the grate and the descending pipe is a door, fastened down, which may be opened, to take out any thing which may be pushed through the grating, before it gets to the descending pipe. Attached to the door of the closet is a spring, which, every time the door is opened, acts upon a valve, connected with a water cistern, from which a large rush of water immediately passes through the trough. An S trap is fixed to the descending pipe in the same way as described above. In addition to these contrivances, to keep the building sweet, all the drains attached to it ought to be of an extra large size, with a good fall ; for, after every precaution, the patients do, and will contrive to cram things into them.

In asylums designed for paupers only, it is unnecessary to have any plaster on the walls ; lime-wash on the bricks is all that is required ; it is easily applied, whenever and wherever it is wanted : in a short time, indeed, it forms of itself such a covering over the bricks, that the absence of the plaster is not observed; and in a large building the saving of money is considerable. The doors, both of the galleries and rooms, should be made substantially strong; none of them panelled. Doors of this description are burst open, by a madman, without the slightest difficulty. As it sometimes happens that a patient will get his bedstead to the door of his cell, and thus barricade the entrance, it would be convenient for some of the doors to open outwards instead of inwards: these may be protected, by bolts, from being forced open from the inside. The plan usually adopted, of having the window-frames made of iron, and the windows small, is a sufficient protection against the patients getting out through them; and the prison-like appearance of iron bars is avoided. The sleeping rooms for the refractory patients should be fitted up with shutters, and it would be convenient for these to be made to slide within the walls: the windows in the refractory galleries should be protected with a wire net-work. Much inconvenience will be experienced if the locks are not on a good principle: they ought to be strong, and of a simple construction; and, if made with the pin to go into the key, it should not be made so large as to weaken the key: keys made so as to admit the pin are very apt to break. One key should open all the locks in the male wards, and another all those in the female wards.

It has been already stated, that the best situation for the kitchen, and all the domestic offices, is at the back of the centre; and this should be their place, whatever be the size of the building. The plan of having two kitchens, one for the males, and another for the females, is perfectly ridiculous: it would necessarily create the necessity of having a double set of servants, and double minor offices of every description, and would greatly increase the labour of the superintendents. This error was unfortunately committed both in the Wakefield and Middlesex Asylums; the consequence has been, that one kitchen at each place is appropriated to other purposes: and the other kitchen, in which all the provisions for both sides of the house are obliged to be cooked, being at one corner of the building, is very inconveniently situated. This would of course be obviated, if the kitchen were placed in the centre. From what has already been stated, relative to the employment of the patients in the different domestic concerns, it will be obvious that the offices should be of ample size. Where the cooking, washing, baking, &c. are all done by the patients, instead of being done by hired servants, of course a greatly increased number of persons will be employed in these works; and, to prevent their interfering with each other, abundant room is required. These offices ought to be double the size that it would be requisite for them to be built if sane persons only were employed. It is particularly desirable for them all, in the first instance, to be rather too large for the number intended to be admitted, as there is scarcely an asylum in the kingdom which has not required enlargement, to meet the wants of the insane, whose numbers augment as the population increases. Another very material consideration is, the ventilation and warming : one mode is by admitting the atmosphere through a tunnel under ground, and then passing it over plates of heated iron, and distributing the warm air, by pipes, throughout the building. In the only asylum in which I have seen this plan tried it did not answer ; and the air seems to lose something of its purity and wholesomeness, by being passed over the hot iron. The plan of warming, by hot water passing along pipes, in the same manner as many hot-houses are warmed, may be conveniently used in small buildings ; but it does not answer when the water has to traverse a considerable distance of piping before it returns to the boiler. As the whole of the water contained in the boiler and pipes must be heated, before sufficient warmth can be produced, too much time is occupied in getting the hot water into circulation : I am, however, by no means certain that a complete apparatus of this kind, for each ward, would not be the most desirable, the most economical, and the most efficient mode of heating the building : it would also be attended with this great advantage, that the heat could be completely regulated, according to the different wants of the patients. Where the whole building is heated by one or two apparatuses, the wards through which the pipes first pass receive a greater portion of heat than is required, and there is great difficulty in keeping the temperature sufficiently high in those which are at the extremities of the building; wherein are usually placed the dirty and imbecile patients, who really require the greatest degree of warmth. Pipes heated by steam, and passing under the floor of the galleries, after many experiments, appear the readiest and best mode of heating any very extended building, by one or two apparatuses. Mr. Bramah has recently invented a plan to exclude the heat, at pleasure, from the wards through which the pipes pass: a pipe is laid under the floor of each ward, along the side of the range of sleeping apartments, in a covered brick air-passage, sufficiently large to admit, from the external atmosphere, as much air as is required for the purposes of ventilation; openings are made in the sides of the cells towards the wards, three or four inches above the floor, capable of being closed, either partially or entirely, by an iron slide. It is expected that this arrangement will obviate the objection, of having the wards near the apparatus too hot, whilst those at a distance from it are not sufficiently heated. Where the building is large, and more than one or two heating apparatuses cannot, from any circumstances, be fixed, I decidedly prefer steam to warm water. Upon a trial of the two plans at the asylum at Hanwell, it was found that the pipes heated by steam attained the temperature of two hundred degrees of Fahrenheit in an hour and a half; and eight hours elapsed before the same length of pipes, heated by hot water, reached the temperature of one hundred and thirty degrees. One objection has been made to the use of steam, which at first appears considerable; it is, that the joints are continually giving way, and the apartments consequently wet and uncomfortable. This is easily obviated by making all the joints with iron-cement, instead of cotton and paint, which are too frequently used. In long ranges of pipes there should be one made of wrought iron, and considerably bent, into the shape of almost two-thirds of a common oval, four feet long : this will allow of the expansion and contraction of the pipes, when heating and cooling. Another great advantage of the heating by steam is, that in an asylum containing three hundred patients, not more than one steam boiler need be in use at the same time : if of a proper size it will warm all the building, heat the water for the washing, and the water in the cisterns in the roof, and heat the drying closets, and also supply all the cooking apparatus with steam. Though it must be admitted that a considerable quantity of coal is consumed by the one boiler, yet, as no fires will be wanted in the wards, the plan is thought rather to diminish than to increase the expense of fuel. When proper care is taken to secure due ventilation, it has one very great advantage over the open fire; which is, that all the patients, the weak as well as the strong, are placed upon an equal footing with respect to warmth. With open fires, when secured by proper guards, all the space round and near them is occupied in cold weather, by the patients least requiring extra warmth;

and the feeble, and those whose circulation is most languid, are pushed away: quarrels and blows are not unfrequent, as may be supposed, under such circumstances; nor can these evils be prevented, unless the attention of one keeper is entirely devoted to watching the fire-place.

When all the patients who can be trusted are kept in regular employment, the airing courts, attached to the different wards, need not be so large or so numerous as is generally thought necessary; two or three at the most, for each sex, will be sufficient. In fine weather, the farm and the garden ought to be the airing courts for the healthy, and in wet weather they must remain within-doors. One airing court for each sex should be larger than the other, and the walls sufficiently high to prevent one patient being able to assist another to escape. In all establishments there will be found some, whose contrivances to accomplish this purpose, and whose dexterity in carrying it into execution, are surprising; and, notwithstanding the greatest vigilance, they often succeed. For such cases there remains only the alternative, of either keeping them constantly locked up, which would be injurious to their health, or having the airing-court walls so high as to be inaccessible. The corners ought not to be rectangular; for, though it does not frequently happen, I have had patients under my care, who could get up to the top of a wall by the square angles, with the aid only of their elbows and knees. The walls of the other courts need not exceed ten feet, and the division walls may be still lower. In each of the courts there should be an awning to protect the patients from the sun. In all institutions for paupers, workshops should be provided, in which the patients may perform different branches of mechanical labour, to which they have previously been accustomed; but, where the apparatus is very expensive, and the labour not likely to be useful to the institution, or profitable, the patient may, by kind perseverance, be induced to learn some mechanical art, which he had never previously attempted. At the asylum at Hanwell, there are no less than six shoemakers now at work, who never did any thing of the kind before their admission; and three, who have been discharged cured, also learnt the trade during their residence in the asylum. Spinning of twine and rope-making are also generally liked; many of the patients prefer them to any other occupation, and they have all been taught to do these works at the asylum. The awnings before spoken of, as shelter from the sun in the airing courts, ought to be sufficiently long to permit these works to be carried on under them. It will be unnecessary to enter more fully into an abstract account of Pauper Lunatic Asylums, as it is proposed to give a description of the one at Hanwell, and to point out how far it does not accord with our views, in those details which remain to be noticed. An account of the mode in which it is actually conducted, will be combined with this description, and form the best commentary on

the chapter on Treatment. The Plan at the commencement of the work shows the situation of the
building : it stands on an estate of about fifty-five
acres, of which the subsoil is gravel; and is beautifully situated on the rise of a hill about eight miles
and a half from London, with its front at a distance
of two hundred and fifty yards to the south of the
Uxbridge road, which forms the northern boundary
of the estate : the river Brent is the eastern boundary ; a farm of the Earl of Jersey the western ; and
the Grand Junction Canal, which communicates with
a dock on the premises, the southern. The whole
estate is abundantly supplied with water. The principal part of the building is two stories high : the
portion between the two dotted lines is that which
was originally built. It was designed for three hundred patients ; but, with greatly economizing the
room, and making use of a part of the basement, it
has been fitted so as to accommodate six hundred
and fifteen. The part of the building on the outer
sides of the dotted lines has been recently built for
the reception of three hundred additional patients.
The entire front from east to west, including the
new part, is nine hundred and ninety-six feet in
length.

It will be observed that the central part of the
building projects a little beyond each of the side
galleries : the length of this projection is thirty-four
feet, and the length of the similar projection of the
side galleries, to the south of the centre of the

building, is also thirty-four feet;* the whole length of
the central part of the building, with its lateral pro-
jections, is five hundred and seventy-six feet; the
extreme length of each of the side galleries, which
run from north to south, including the tower and
abutment, is three hundred and sixty-two feet.
There is in the centre, and also in each of the side
wings, an octagonal tower, eighty feet in diameter,
and three stories high; each side of which is thirty-
four feet long. Thus it will be seen that a small
wing, which is two stories high, is carried out from the
south side of the central tower; this wing is thirty-
four feet long. Previous to the recent addition to the
building, the wings, springing from the side towers,
were of the same dimensions; the new portion
added to each is one hundred and eighty-seven feet
long. The transverse part, at each of the extremities of the new building, is three stories high; and
extends from north to south seventy-five feet. The
principal entrance is in the front tower, which contains the committee-room, the superintendent and
matron's apartments, with domestic offices, the
chapel, and the day rooms or dining rooms of a
male and female ward. On the east of this tower
are the wards for the male, on the west those for
the female patients: the old building contains fifteen
of these wards, seven for the males and eight for the

* I am indebted to the Clerk of the Works for the New Building for these measurements; I have therefore no doubt of their
accuracy.

females; the numbers in each vary from twenty-six to sixty. Each of the wards consists of a gallery ten feet wide, and ten feet and a half high, with sleeping apartments on the side of it looking towards the building, the other side affording a cheerful view into the surrounding country. In the new building there are sleeping apartments on both sides of the galleries, but openings are left abundantly sufficient for light and air, and they are intended to be principally occupied by violent patients. A day room, in which the patients dine, is also attached to each of the wards in the old building; in the new building the openings in the galleries will be used for that purpose. The western octagonal tower contains the apartments for the surgeon and sub-matron, with a waiting and receiving room, and dining and sleeping rooms for the insane: the bazaar also is in a room in this tower. The eastern tower is appropriated to the residence of the surgeon, who, when the new building is occupied, will be appointed more immediately to attend to the male patients: it also contains the surgery and office. In the basement of this tower are the shops for the joiners, painters, glaziers, brush-makers, and coopers: there are staircases from the top to the bottom of the house in each of the octagonal towers; and there is also one at each corner of the central part of the building; there are also smaller staircases communicating from the wards to the airing court. The situation and size of the airing courts are sufficiently pointed out in the engraving. The two portions of the building in a line with the wings, running from north to south, which project beyond the southern front of the building, were originally designed to be used as kitchens for the two sides of the house; but as the having two kitchens would have increased the number of the servants, and would also have been attended with additional expense and trouble, the portion of the building intended for the western kitchen has been altered into a ward, so as to accommodate a considerable number of patients, and the cooking for the establishment is entirely carried on in the eastern kitchen.

This is forty-five feet long, by thirty-four wide, externally. It contains four steam-tables, two steam-boilers, a stew hearth, a common kitchen cooking grate, with the necessary tables, drawers and binns for salt, rice, oatmeal, &c. Contiguous to it is the scullery, fitted up with the usual appendages and coppers for boiling vegetables. The dairy and larder are conveniently situated in ample cellars near the kitchen. At the back of the kitchen and scullery is a closed yard, around the sides of which are the bake-house, brew-house, poultry-house, gas-house, and the house for the boiler, which supplies the cooking apparatus with steam, and heats the eastern side of the building; there is also a large bath, with proper apparatus for filling it either with hot or cold water. Around a yard similarly situated on the western side of the house, are placed the wash-house, drying closets, laundry, and foul-linen room. This yard is used for drying linen out of doors when the weather will permit : the wash-house is seventy-three and a half feet long, by twenty-five wide, externally, and furnished with fixed washing-tubs, into which hot and cold water is conveyed by taps. It is filled with large wooden steeping-troughs, and with a most useful washing-machine, worked by steam power upon the principle of a fulling-mill. It also contains an hydraulic press, which squeezes out the water from the clothes with much less injury to the fabric, and less labour than the hand wringing. It is not thought that these fitments can be improved. The drying closet is seven feet six inches high, to the wall plate, twenty-two feet nine inches long, and eleven feet two inches wide. It is heated by steam-pipes, and furnished with an opening at the top for the passage of the condensed vapour thrown off from the wet clothes. The laundry is fifty-nine and a half feet long, and twenty-five feet wide, externally; it contains a large ironing-board, extending the whole length of the room, various tables, an ironing stove, two mangles on the rotatory principle, and a smaller drying closet for the purpose of completely airing the clothes. The wash-house and drying closet for wet sheets, and other foul linen, are, at Hanwell, as they ought to be in all asylums, detached from the general wash-house. This wash-house is fitted up with a common washing-machine; and whatever be the state of the weather, wet mattresses and clothes are exposed to the atmosphere, previously to being completely dried in the closet. In this yard is also placed the store room, a repository for the clothing and other articles; and it contains a bath for the females similar to that already described. Behind this yard, and at a short distance from the wash-house, are placed the steam-engine and the house containing its boiler, and another for the production of steam to supply the laundry and dry closets, and also to warm the western side of the building. Adjacent is the blacksmith's shop, with a lathe; and a few feet from it is the tinner's workshop. The engraving will show the situation of the dock; around it are coal-sheds. The cow-house, piggery, and stables are conveniently placed at the back of the house. There are two kitchen gardens: the one on the east side of the house contains upwards of four acres; the other, which is at the south-western corner of the estate, appears in the engraving, enclosed with two walks at right angles to each other, and with a curvilinear wall. This curvilinear wall, extending four hundred and seventy-five feet in length and ten feet in height, was entirely built by the patients; it contains about two acres and three quarters.

We must now, in pursuance of our plan, give an account of the mode in which the Asylum at Hanwell is actually managed. The detail will be to many uninteresting; but it is hoped that it may suggest useful hints to those about to undertake the superintendence of similar institutions.

The Asylum, having been erected according to the provisions of the act of parliament, 9 Geo. IV., is necessarily under the management of a Committee of county magistrates: this consists of fifteen members, five of whom go out every year, but are eligible to be re-elected. The times of their holding meetings are uncertain, varying with the business to be transacted: when any thing particular is going forward, or is wanted, they are held as often as once in a week or fortnight: in the winter season they usually take place at the Sessions House, Clerkenwell. From April to September, a meeting is always held on the second Monday in every month at the Asylum, in addition to those held at the Sessions House, for entering into contracts for provisions, coals, &c. every three months: independently of these regular meetings for business, the members of the committee, particularly those residing in the neighbourhood of the Asylum, are in the habit of very frequently visiting it at uncertain times, and inspecting sometimes a part, sometimes the whole of the building: a plan that cannot be too much commended and imitated. These visits are of much more importance to the real well-being of the establishment, than those which take place at regular and stated periods; they ought never to be relaxed, even if good order and propriety be uniformly found in every department. They will

always afford gratification to those who do their
duty, when made in the usual spirit and manner
practised by gentlemen, who are in general appointed
county magistrates ; and they are a great incentive
to activity to those who might be disposed to be
negligent if entirely freed from such useful inspection.   They are also very much calculated to
strengthen the hands of the Superintendents.   The
subordinate officers and servants, knowing that the
members of the committee are in the habit of going
round the Asylum, will. be kept alert, and attention
and diligence, on their parts, will be the result.

Once a quarter the books and accounts of the
establishment are very carefully examined ; any two
or three of the gentlemen, who may happen to be
present, assisting the chairman to inspect them, and
compare the bills and vouchers for the articles procured since the last examination.   A statement is
then laid before them of such things as are expected
to be wanted before the next meeting : they give
their orders for these in writing, their own clerk
being in attendance to take down the transactions
of the meeting.

The execution of the different orders made by the
committee is entrusted to the resident medical superintendent, a physician, and the matron, who are man
and wife.   When the peculiar circumstances of these
establishments are taken into consideration, it seems
a most desirable arrangement that the direction of
them should be in the hands of married persons ; it

gives a home feeling to the parties, and prevents the little petty quarrelling and jealousies which are found continually to exist where single persons preside, and each has a separate interest to attend to. These officers have the entire management, under the control of the committee, of the details of the institution, and give the orders for such things as they have received instructions for from the committee, and for any works of necessity that may arise. The medical and moral treatment of all the patients is under the immediate direction of the resident physician and matron : the resident physician also acts as the treasurer to the institution. The resident physician and matron are assisted by the house surgeon and his wife ; the former of whom, immediately after the patients have breakfasted, goes round the wards on both sides of the house, and carefully examines into the state and general health and comfort of the patients, and makes a report of any new case of sickness to the physician, whom he subsequently accompanies in his rounds : he also makes up the medicines, and keeps the medical case-book. In the afternoon this officer again regularly goes round the wards ; in fact, his duty consists in the exercising a constant watchfulness over the servants, particularly over the male keepers, and in the becoming intimately acquainted with the character and circumstances of each individual patient, so as to contrive, with the physician and matron, that not an opportunity may be lost of taking advantage of any favourable turn in the disease. This duty is unceasing; it embraces occasional visits, at uncertain times, to the different male wards, before the servants rise in the morning, to see that the keepers do not permit the patients to get up before they themselves are dressed and ready to attend them, and similar visits after the patients are put to-bed at night; to take care that the patients' clothes are taken out of their bed-rooms; and that the epileptic patients are so secured as to be unable to turn upon the face, without which precaution they are liable to die from suffocation, in case of a fit coming on. It of course also embraces an attendance, in conjunction with the physician, on any special cases of sickness, as often as may be needed. This officer and the clerk, in each week, inspect the stock of linen, bedding, clothes, &c. in each of the male wards; and, comparing it with the inventory, report any deficiency to the matron. When the institution receives the additional number of three hundred patients, which it has been recently enlarged to contain, an additional house surgeon will be appointed, who will have under his charge the male patients; and the attention of Dr. Button, the present house surgeon, will be more particularly confined to the females. A consulting physician and consulting surgeon are appointed, who render their services in cases of difficulty and emergency, and whenever the committee of visiting magistrates think necessary.

The wife of the house surgeon, in the first place,

takes care that the female sick are properly and kindly attended to; that the medicines and food ordered for them are duly administered : she also attends to the general comfort of the female wards, and minutely examines into the state of the beds, linen, &c. .She also sees that the regulations given to the female keepers are complied with, and takes care that no permission of absence is given which would leave any particular department without a due number of female attendants. This is easily arranged, as no servant is allowed to go out of the lodge gate without a pass ticket, signed by the superintendent, and left at the lodge, and brought up the next morning by the porter for inspection. To her is entrusted the distribution of the pass tickets to the female servants. She also takes care that the breakfasts and dinners for the females are of good quality, and sufficient in quantity, and that they are duly distributed according to the proper rations for each ward. The afternoon is spent by her amongst the female wards, and she assists in carrying out the little plans formed by the physician and matron, for the employment and moral treatment of the females; and she communicates to them any information which, from conversation with the patients, or with their friends, or from any other source, she may think likely to be valuable. After the female patients have gone to bed, during each week, she examines one-third of the bed-rooms : this examination takes place at uncertain times. A similar examination is made of the other bed-rooms by the workwoman and the female store-keeper. The store-keeper and Mrs. Button take the stock of the female wards every week. The clerk to the institution keeps the various books of account relating to the receipts and disbursements of the establishment, and to the ordering and receipt of goods from the various tradesmen. No orders for goods are permitted to be sent to any tradesman without the express authority of the superintendent or matron for each individual article. Every Tuesday morning, at nine o'clock, the officers and the keeper from each ward, who is entrusted with the mechanical work carried on by the patients in it, and one of the female nurses from each ward, meet the superintendent and matron in the committee room, and give an account of the work which has been executed under their direction during the past week, and receive instructions as to their employment until the next meeting ; and they mention the various articles which are wanted, and such of them as on inquiry and examination are ascertained to be proper, are ordered by the superintendent and matron.   The clerk enters their orders into the order book, and on the arrival of the goods they are carefully examined ; the invoice, if correct, copied, and a receipt corresponding with the copied invoice is given to the tradesman.   No goods are received without such an invoice ; and, on the coming in of the tradesmen's bills, each item charged is carefully checked with the copies of the invoices.   The clerk also keeps the books relating to the patients, and examines and files the warrants and certificates which are sent with them on their admission; and receives orders from the house surgeon as to the ward to which each patient is to be sent. If the patient be a female, he furnishes an account in writing of the particulars mentioned in the warrant, and the house surgeon endeavours to procure from the overseers, or the friends who accompany the patient, such information as may be useful in the treatment. The clerk also takes care that the male side of the house, and the outer doors are properly secured with the master-key at the conclusion of the evening prayers.

In contemplation of the additional number of patients, a provision store-keeper is appointed. He receives the meat from the butcher, and sees that it is of due weight and quality, and immediately reports any deficiencies in either respect. The receipt of the groceries is also entrusted to him; and the daily weighing the provisions, and the distributing the raw material, by weight and measure, to a part of the *manufactories*, also falls to his duty; and however unappropriate such a term might appear, when applied to lunatics, it is strictly correct, and the attending to it occupies a considerable portion of time; for manufactures are carried on by the patients, and to a great extent; and the hemp for the band and twine-spinning, the coir for the teasing, the leather for the shoe-making, the pottle-wood for the pottle-making, the straw for the hat-making, the willows for basket-making, bristles for brush-making, are duly given out by measure, and accurate note is taken of the quantity of the material used, and of the manufactured article returned. This officer also takes care that the conduct of the servant in the kitchen is orderly and respectable.

The housekeeper takes care that the female servants, in her department, are in due time in the morning at work with their patients. She receives the milk for the breakfasts of the patients, and sees that they are duly prepared according to the diet-table, a copy of which will be found in the Appendix. She has the entire responsibility of the cooking for the patients and officers. Her only sane assistant in the kitchen is the dairy-maid, when not engaged in her milking and other duties. She has also the distribution of the butter, bread, and such other of the provisions as are not under the keeping of the provision store-keeper. In the evening she takes care that the domestic servants, with such of the patients as remain up to help them, attend the family prayers, which are regularly held in the chapel at half past nine.

The female store-keeper has under her charge the entire stock in hand of all the clothing and bedding for the men and women, not given out to the keepers and nurses of the respective wards; and in each week she takes an account of all the linen wanting repair. This she receives from the laundry-maid, and provides for its being duly repaired in the female wards, and out of her stores substitutes other articles in good order. She also receives the bread and groceries for the females, in bulk, from the provision store-keeper, and duly apportions them; and in like manner she duly apportions to the respective female nurses, the articles for the employment of their patients, and collects them and takes an account of them in detail when manufactured. Every morning and afternoon, she collects the female patients, to be employed in out-door work, and sends them, under the charge of proper female nurses, to the gardener, with a written paper containing their numbers. He employs them, under the care of the nurse, in such portion of the out-door work as may be desirable; and the female store-keeper, each morning and afternoon, visits the females at work out of doors, and takes care that they are properly attended to by the nurse, under whose immediate charge they are placed. She gives out such of the stores under her care as are wanted for the week's consumption, and examines and compares the goods, previous to their being deposited in her room, with the nurses; and gives the clerk a written acknowledgment of having received them, and duly enters them in her account-book : and no articles are given out of her room without an account of them being also kept. By this means the entire stock of articles in the house can be immediately ascertained. The store-keeper, with the assistance of the patients, cuts out all the linen for the house and patients; she also has the charge of the patients' library, for which they are principally indebted to the kindness of Mr.

Gurney. It consists of interesting biography, voyages, travels, short historical accounts of different parts, and amusing anecdotes. These, with tracts, are distributed every Saturday amongst the different keepers, for the use of the patients for the ensuing week ; or are lent to the individual patients, at their personal request; and an account of them is carefully kept. A copy of the Penny and Saturday Magazine is also taken in by the Institution, for the use of the patients. The library is a source of great amusement; and as the books are distributed on Saturday, the reading them sometimes to one another, sometimes alone, serves to occupy the mind, and keep the patients quiet on Sunday—by far the most difficult day in the week to manage them. The patients, on that day not having their ordinary employment, and not being previously accustomed to amuse themselves with mental occupations, suffer from *ennui;* and the result of their idleness is a greater quantity of vice and mischief on that day than on any other in the week.

In the afternoon the men and women assemble together in the chapel, and practise singing the hymns and psalms which are to form a part of the evening services : but as the singing takes up a considerable portion of the afternoon, of course it is not confined to these. At six o'clock in the evening, Dr. Stoddard, the chaplain, performs divine service, and there is as much anxiety amongst the patients to be permitted to attend, and to come in their best dresses, as there is amongst the sane, previous to an attendance on the most fashionable congregation in London; and it would be difficult to find in the metropolis one more orderly or devout. In fact, from the chaplain only attending once on the Sunday, the privilege of being permitted to join in the worship conducted by him is more valued, than if he performed the service more frequently : and the effect upon the patients is, I think, better than if it were less estimated, as it would be if there were more frequent opportunities of enjoying it. The chaplain very judiciously varies the portions of the prayers selected for the service, which he does not permit to extend much above an hour and a quarter. This is quite as long as their attention can be profitably occupied ; and by this arrangement the patients become acquainted with the whole of the Liturgy. The chaplain, once each quarter, administers the sacrament, and many of the patients derive great consolation from being partakers of this ordinance.

The female workwoman is a very important person in the institution ; every alternate week she relieves the female store-keeper of the distribution before breakfast of the bread and groceries : after breakfast she is always employed in cutting out, arranging, superintending the making, and selling the various articles, which are to be disposed of in the bazaar. Many of the patients in the Asylum at Hanwell have been reduced to pauperism solely from their insanity ; and others of them have been

in the habit of employing themselves in fine needle-
work. A considerable difficulty was felt in finding
suitable occupation for such patients; the ordinary
sewing and mending, which were wanted for the
institution, were disliked, and there appeared no
means of procuring for them work suited to their
tastes. With a view to obviate the evils of idleness
in this class, the matron hit upon the plan of establishing a bazaar. She borrowed of the treasurer
twenty-three pounds eighteen shillings : this she
laid out in the purchase of a few articles in the first
instance as patterns, and in the buying the requisite
materials. These are made up and worked by the
patients, and sold by the workwoman to visitors at
the bazaar, or are sent off to order. The scheme
has answered beyond the most sanguine expecta-
tions. At the end of the first year, the whole
amount borrowed from the treasurer, was returned
out of the profits of the sale of the goods; and the
matron was left with a small stock on hand, and
with money due to her. The plan has been persevered
in, and the workwoman has now between forty and
fifty female patients, daily employed in the making
useful and fancy articles for sale. The greatest
difficulty was felt, in the first instance, in obtaining
a market for the goods. But as they are good and
cheap of the kind, this obstacle is gradually being
overcome. It is hardly possible to conceive the
benefit which the patients have derived from this
employment : it is congenial to their previous habits,

it excites a great interest; many of them select and contrive with as much anxiety the various patterns, as if they were exclusively to derive all the profit from their sale. One poor woman who had been insane a long time previous to her admission in 1831, and who was subject to frequent and violent paroxysms, and whom no persuasion could previously induce to work on the establishment of the bazaar, spent her time in minutely working collars and ladies' dresses. This employment was of her own selection, and it so absorbed her attention that the irritability by degrees wore off; and after having for a long time past exhibited no symptom of insanity, she was discharged cured. Others take the charge of particular portions of the work, and employ under them patients, with less mental powers than themselves. In fact there have been many contrivances for the happy occupation of the patients, but I do not think that any have been more beneficial to them than the bazaar. In a pecuniary point of view, the speculation has been very profitable. An exact account is kept of the cost of every article used, from the pins upwards, and of the produce of the sale of the goods. The details of them are furnished to the matron every Saturday by the workwoman. The matron then duly enters these in her book, the bazaar account being kept totally distinct from the other accounts of the institution. At the end of the second year, the profits have enabled the committee, out of them, to purchase an organ for the patients. The instrument is most excellent; it is a complete finger organ, perfect in all its notes, and of beautiful workmanship. It is also fitted with barrels capable of playing twenty-four tunes. As it is principally intended to assist in divine service, the music set upon the barrels is sacred; but the patients assemble one evening in each week to enjoy a little concert. The patients, by the profits of whose labour the organ has been purchased, and others equally industrious, though in another way, who take an interest in the musical performances, have been consulted on the selection of the tunes: this creates an interest in them about the organ, and the establishment generally, which it is very desirable to keep up; it adds a little too to their self-respect, and raises them in the moral scale; and God forbid that the time should ever arrive when any thing, little or great, should be neglected, which would tend to soothe their feelings, or to make less bitter the nauseous, though necessary cup of confinement! The musical meetings are looked forward to with great pleasure. A similar plan was, and still is, adopted at Wakefield. I remember one of the patients there, an exceedingly violent man, who was obliged to be kept almost constantly in confinement, on whom the music had such an influence, that on being allowed to attend, which was permitted at his request and promise of good behaviour, he always conducted himself with the greatest propriety: unfortunately, neither the promise nor the good behaviour extended after the time of his return to his ward. In his case the insanity was, as far as I remember, brought on by a blow on the head; and I have no doubt, that organic disease in the brain was the cause of his violence, which was, however, suspended by the "concord of sweet sounds." The patients, who are attached to the bazaar, are not permitted to remain in the house during the whole day; but they are sent out, in many cases much against their inclinations, when the weather is fine, for a short time every morning and after-noon, into the grounds; where they assist in any work which does not require much muscular strength. This has a great tendency to keep them in health. It is hoped that the profits of the bazaar will be exclusively appropriated to the increase of the comforts of the patients.

It has been already stated that the building is heated by steam. The water is pumped into a cistern in the roof by a steam-engine, which also works the washing machine previously described. The whole of the machinery is under the charge of an engineer: he regulates the temperature of the wards by adjusting the admission of the proper quantity of steam. Much of his time is occupied in repairing and keeping the machinery in order: he also takes charge of the stock of iron, and of the blacksmith's shop. He is assisted by the fireman, who attends to the various boilers, and works, with two or three patients under his charge, in the blacksmith's shop.

There are two gardeners. The head gardener is responsible for the finding of the vegetables which are required by the housekeeper, to whom he delivers, by weight and measure, each day's consumption: he also keeps an account of all the male and female patients who go out to work, and he is responsible for their safe return: he apportions their work to them, and takes care that each set of patients shall be under the charge of proper persons. He is principally occupied in the eastern garden; the assisting gardener attends more particularly to the western. He receives from the head gardener a number of male and female patients, with their names, who are employed under his direction. The supply of vegetables is abundant.

The cropping and cultivating the parts of the land not included in the gardens devolves upon the farming man: he also has the management of the cows and pigs. He is assisted by a number of male patients, for whom he is accountable whilst they are under his employment: this number varies, according to circumstances, from twelve to forty. He has also the help of a carter, who delivers the coals from the sheds, when they are landed at the dock side, to the different offices. He also goes to London once a week with a cart, to fetch the goods ordered for the use of the institution. This arrangement effects a considerable saving to the establishment. There are usually about fifty-five male and thirty-three female patients employed in gardening and farming.

A dairy-maid, with her staff of from four to six female patients, assists the farming-man in the milking. The 612 patients, now in the house, daily consume the milk of about sixteen cows: she also assists the housekeeper in the kitchen, and in the taking up and apportioning the dinners.

The bread and beer of the establishment are made by one sane female, assisted by eight patients. The regularity of the system laid down for her enables this servant to accomplish the whole of the baking and brewing for the 660 persons, of whom the family now consists.

The washing for the 612 patients and servants is managed by one laundry-maid, who has under her charge from sixteen to twenty patients. Their time is, as may be supposed, sufficiently occupied by the washing and getting up the linen of all the patients, servants, and officers in the establishment.

There are two keepers to each ward, one of whom is a mechanic. Before breakfast, both are employed in getting up, washing, and shaving the patients. After breakfast, the one, who is a mechanic, leaves the ward in charge of the other; and he selects from his own ward, and from the other male wards, such patients as are able to work with him at his trade, and whom the superintendent and surgeon may think proper to be entrusted to him. These patients either go with him to his shop, or are employed about the building, wherever their services may be wanted. The keeper who is left in the ward, attends to the patients, takes care that the beds are made, the rooms and gallery thoroughly cleaned, and employs the patients in picking coir, twine-spinning, or any other in-door employment, which is carried on in his ward.

Each female ward has two nurses : at nine o'clock the junior nurse, whenever the weather permits, collects those patients in her ward who are to be employed out of doors, and assists and watches over them whilst in the cultivation of the ground. The necessary ward duties, mending the clothes for the male and female patients, the making the whole of the house linen, and assisting in sewing the men's clothes (cut out by the tailor), the superintending the twine-spinning, basket-making, pottle-making and other works, carried on in the wards, afford sufficient occupation to the nurse who is left in charge of it. In the Appendix will be found a copy of the Rules which apply to the keepers and nurses.

Each parish has the privilege of sending into the institution a number of patients, in proportion to the sum contributed by it to the building the Asylum ; the cost of which, including cost of the fifty-five acres of land, and of the furnishing, and also law and all other expenses, was 124,456l. 14s. 5d. As the Asylum has long been quite full, it unfortunately happens, that a long time frequently elapses before patients can be received, after the application for their admission. The days for their reception are Tuesdays and Fridays, between the hours of eleven

and one. On the arrival of each patient, the warrant for his admission is seen to be correct, and
inquiries are made of the overseers and friends, in
order to obtain such information as may enable the
surgeon to select the most appropriate ward, and to
warn the keeper or nurse, in case of there being any
disposition to violence or suicide. After the ward
has been chosen, the patient is entrusted to the
keeper or nurse, and is immediately stripped, thoroughly cleaned, and clothed in the asylum dress.
The clothes in which the patient comes, are taken
away by the overseer. The patient is seen in the
afternoon by the house surgeon, who ascertains the
general state of the health, and, if requisite, calls in
the advice of the physician : if not, on accompanying the physician in his rounds, on the next morning,
he reports the case to him, and the patient is examined by them, and the moral and medical treatment prescribed. If the case be recent, the plan
previously pointed out is according to the varying
circumstances adopted, and this necessarily prevents
the patient from immediately falling into the ordinary
course pursued, where nearly all are old and incurable
cases. But if the case be, as it generally turns out,
an old case, after a few days' careful watching, in
order to ascertain the peculiarities of the patient, an
attempt is made to induce him to employ himself,
and to become, as it were, one of the family. The
chapter on Treatment has already developed the
principle on which these attempts are made. The

superintendent usually examines the head of the patient phrenologically, and forms his own conjectures as to the character : but he never allows this examination to lead to any diminution of caution ; although, in many cases, the conformation of the head induces the use of beneficial means, which would not have been suggested from any information received with the patient ; this is generally very defective. In the first instance, out-of-door employment is generally tried ; the patient is put under the especial charge of one of the servants, and set to work on the ground in such a way as to avoid any danger of his injuring himself or others. By-and-by, as his character becomes more known, and it is considered safe to trust him, in case of his being a mechanic, he is taken to the keeper, who has the same occupation with which he is acquainted, and is induced to work at his trade. And as there are bricklayers, joiners, tinners, blacksmiths, shoemakers, tailors, brushmakers, twine-makers, pottle-makers, basket-makers and coopers, all at work about the institution, it is most probable that a mechanic will be able to select from amongst them some occupation with which he has been previously acquainted, or which he may like to learn : at all events, the reward of a little tea, tobacco, beer, or some other luxury, congenial to his taste, will, with a little management, generally be sufficient to induce him to occupy himself, either in his ward or out of doors. Indeed, on an average, 454 patients, out of the

612, are daily employed : and of the others, who are idle, some are fatuous, others in such a state of debility as to be unable to work, and only very few idle solely from disinclination to employment. The patients rise at six in the morning, at eight they assemble in the chapel for family prayers, and immediately afterwards they breakfast. At nine they go to their work ; at eleven the workers out of doors have an allowance of one-third of a pint of beer ; at one they dine ; at four they have a similar allowance of beer ; and at seven they sup. Each patient goes into the warm bath, for a thorough washing, every week.

It will be unnecessary to add, that the keeping in order so complex a machine, even now that its parts are carefully arranged, requires the constant and anxious watchful attention of the superintendent and matron : there is not a single movement which does not directly emanate from them. Not a single article is permitted to be ordered without their express direction, and from them, individually, has originated each of the various occupations which are now carried on in the institution, to the comfort and happiness of the patients. The selecting the proper agents to assist them in accomplishing their design has been one of their most difficult tasks. If the choice and dismissal of these agents had not been entrusted to them, it would have been impossible that the present system could have been carried into execution : a minute personal attention is required for the success of it, which can only be ensured by the personal superintendence of those who are immediately in authority. Many little things, the neglect of any one of which could not be made to appear to a committee as a sufficient ground for the dismissal of an officer or servant, are essential to the comfort of the patients; and some of these are in themselves so irksome, that nothing but the knowledge that the disregard of any orders, which affect the welfare of the patients, will at once be followed by some punishment, and, if persisted in, with a dismissal without appeal, can secure diligent and constant attention. It will easily be supposed, that the arranging the details previously pointed out, and the carrying into execution the varied employments of the patients were not accomplished without much labour and anxiety : in the first place, the servants naturally threw every obstacle in the way of their doing any thing; it was much more trouble for the keepers to see that the patients performed the daily necessary household duties, on which their personal comfort in a great measure depended, than it would have been for them to have known, that whether the patients worked or not, their dinners would be cooked, their bread baked, their vegetables gathered by hired sane persons; and of course they would have preferred a sufficient number of sane helpers in the wards to have kept these in order. The having the responsibility of seeing that a much greater portion of work was daily and properly performed than they could individually, however industrious, personally execute, compelled them, but most reluctantly, to call in the assistance of the patients : and at the time when the Asylum was opened, in 1831, the system, which was not at all unusual in many of the poor-houses, of paying its inmates for all the services rendered, created, on the part of the patients, an unwillingness to work ; this, however, was easily overcome. If the patients are in good health, and in a proper state to work, they are allowed no beer, and every little indulgence is withheld, so long as they are idle. They soon find out that employment tends to their comfort ; and when they see those about them happily engaged, and in the enjoyment of the little reward of their industry, they generally very soon petition for something to do. After the prejudices against employing the patients about the house and grounds had in some measure been overcome, there was still an apparently insuperable objection to their making any thing for sale out of the institution. It was said and thought, that the making articles for sale would be an injury to those now employed in them ; and this feeling was not confined to the servants, but it still prevails, and, to a very great degree, amongst the shopkeepers in the metropolis. They, for some reason which I cannot devise, dislike to encourage our attempts : and the store-keeper, who has made inquiries of different tradesmen with a view to the sale of articles manufactured in the asylum, has been

abused as a "thief," for attempting to rob of their
profits those who are now employed in these manufactures ; as if it were possible that the few articles
brought into the market by the labour of the poor
lunatics could really prejudice any one.   If this difficulty had not been overcome it must have put an
end to the plan; as, whatever benefit the patients
might have derived from the labour, this is not the
time when a consideration of their comfort would
counterbalance the most trifling additional expense.
The utilitarian feeling of the present day, which
has no other measure for that which is good and
valuable, than a pecuniary standard, renders it essential that the manufactures should be so carried on as
to be a source not of loss but of profit.   By personal
applications, by letter, by enlisting in the cause of
humanity the active and benevolent, (whose services
I here, on behalf of my poor patients, gratefully
acknowledge,) the labour of the patients has been
rendered available, not only to their own amusement, but to the diminution of their expense, even
after they have been permitted, from the profits,
to enjoy some little comforts which the institution
would not otherwise have provided : these consist
of beer, tea, tobacco, and a variation in the ordinary
dress, or some other indulgence suited to the
tastes of the patients.   Money is, on no account,
permitted to be given them : notwithstanding that
each patient, who fairly gains it, whatever be his
capacity, has his reward, the cost a week for their

board, clothing, medical and other attendance, medicine and washing, and indeed for every expense in any way connected with them, is 5s. 3d.; and I am convinced, that a diminution of their comforts will not be attended with a saving to the institution. Once take away the inducement for them to employ themselves, and you must immensely increase by far the most expensive part of the establishment, the servants; and there would be no little addition to the expense in the injuries which would be done by the patients, by their applying, to mischievous purposes, that muscular or nervous energy, which is now profitably spent in useful labour. It would be tedious to detail the opposition which each new art has met with on its introduction: suffice it to say, that each, without any exception, has at its commencement been thwarted. It has only been by insisting, that whether the servants learnt or not, they should remain with the patients until they might have an opportunity of being taught, and by making a careful selection from amongst the patients to become the pupils, that these manufactures have been successively established. I will only add one observation: hitherto no accident of any consequence has happened from the patients being entrusted with tools, and no unpleasant result has arisen from the female patients, under proper charge of their nurses, working in the grounds or shops, where male patients, also under proper care, have been at the same time employed. And as far as the greatest vigilance and precaution can avail, the benefit of the system, without suffering from any inconveniences to which it is exposed, will continue to be received. It is, however, possible that some untoward accident may happen : but even then I should be sorry for the system to be given up. The injuries, in one or two instances, are nothing in comparison with the constant and daily happiness which it affords to hundreds ; and it is not possible, in this world, to have a great good, without some danger of evil arising from it. But as, in the ordinary events of life, we do not permit a little inconvenience to stand in the way of our enjoying great happiness, so ought we not, in this case, to be deterred from pursuing our plan, even should some unforeseen calamity, which I pray God to forbid, overtake us.

From what has been said on the treatment of the insane in Lunatic Asylums, it will be obvious, that, according to my notions, no one, except a medical man, and a benevolent one, ought to be entrusted with the management of them. I deeply regret, that during the progress of the work, I have learnt that Government have sent out, as the superintendent of the only public asylum in New South Wales, an individual, without any medical education whatever. The only knowledge of the disease possessed by himself and his wife, the matron, has been derived from their being keepers in a private asylum. Now, I have nothing whatever to say in disparagement of the characters of these individuals: so far from it, as far as I could judge of the superintendent, whom I saw at Hanwell, I believe him to have a sincere desire to do good; and I know that he regrets his want of knowledge. But surely there is not in the mighty empire of the south, which must eventually rival in importance, as it now exceeds Europe in extent, such a superabundance of light and knowledge, that a Government, which has its welfare at heart, can afford to throw away an opportunity of establishing on a right principle, of setting up as a model for imitation, an institution for the cure of a disease, to which, it is to be feared, the habits and characters of the inhabitants will render them peculiarly liable. This is not a light matter : the parliamentary investigation in 1815 showed us, that in England, in the midst of medical knowledge, and of a population advanced in morals, intellect and benevolence, there existed in Asylums evils, appalling and revolting to humanity. And by this appointment, Government have set the example of placing these institutions, in a country uninfluenced by moral checks, under the control of a class of persons, entirely unqualified for their management. It is no answer to the objection, that the personal character of the individual appointed will, in the particular hospital, prevent the abuse. The nature of the appointment shows, that, in the opinion of Government, insanity is not a curable disease : and with the sanction of such authority, must we not expect, that asylums, to be built there, will be considered rather as prisons for the safe custody of the insane, than as hospitals for their cure? If this opinion be once generally held, is it reasonable to hope, that there will not occur, in future asylums in New South Wales, scenes rivalling, in wretchedness and infamy, those brought to light in 1815? If such be the case, verily Government will not be guiltless.

CHAPTER IX.

ON THE DISTINCTION BETWEEN CONDUCT WHICH IS
THE RESULT OF MORAL EVIL, AND THAT WHICH
ARISES FROM INSANITY.

HAVING endeavoured to show, that insanity is a
disease of the brain, or nervous system, producing
or accompanied by some injurious alteration in the
intellectual manifestations, or in the conduct, it will
be necessary for us to consider the moral condition
of man in his natural state, independently of any
physical disease, in order that we may not mistake
the consequence of moral evil for derangement,
and refer to mental disorder acts which are really
only the result of vicious propensities.

Whatever be the origin of moral evil, its existence,
both amongst the sane and the insane, is universally
acknowledged. The mode in which it exhibits itself, varies according to the natural character.
Education and the forms of society will do much to
prevent its displaying itself in a way so greatly in_
jurious as to make personal restraint necessary.
Indeed with most, the immediate suffering produced
by a certain measure of vicious indulgence imposes

a limit to the gratification of the natural propensities, whatever these may be : but where the passions
are violent, and the habitual indulgence of them has
been unchecked by education or religion, they gradually become more and more powerful ; and even
where no physical disease exists, acts are committed
so entirely opposite to the feelings of a good and
virtuous man, that he is unable to account for them,
and he attributes them from kind, but mistaken
views, to insanity.   But such acts differ essentially
from those which arise from mental derangement :
they are not the result of any morbid action in the
brain, or nervous system, or of any diseased organization there ; and they are entirely optional.   The
mere fact, that the temporary gratification of the
particular passion is purchased at a most unwise expense of subsequent pain, is no proof of the existence
of insanity.   To a holy man, who feels that he is
constantly in the presence of a God, who " hateth
iniquity," every wilful violation of his laws must,
when calmly considered, be deemed contrary to
right reason.   But it would be perfectly absurd to
characterize every sinful act as an act of madness.
Mankind are too apt to make their own notions of
morals the standard by which they measure the
actions of others, and to consider, that any step
much beyond the bounds, which they have marked
out as the limit within which vice may be indulged
in with comparative impunity, is to be attributed to
insanity.   It is, however, obvious, that a standard

which would vary not only with individuals but with entire nations, furnishes no test that can be depended upon to distinguish between moral evil and derangement. The error arises from the same source, which causes conduct merely eccentric to be considered the result of insanity. We are apt to refer all actions to the test of our individual consciousness; and if we know, that, under similar circumstances, the doing them would be so entirely contrary to our dispositions as to cause us positive pain, we cannot account for them on any reasonable principles, and therefore satisfy ourselves by the conclusion, that the man must be mad. Indeed some, and with greater consistency, go so far as to say that they consider all men, more or less, mad : this, however, is a mere verbal fallacy. The persons who so use the term, know that it is totally inapplicable to any practical purpose, and they admit the necessity of distinguishing between those " mad acts," which deserve to be punished as vicious, and those for which they consider the state of mind of the individual a sufficient excuse. I cannot think that any act, however vicious or eccentric, ought to be considered as the result of insanity, unless it is involuntary, and arising from some disease in the brain or nervous system. In many of the insane, particular sets of feelings and propensities are excited into such undue action, that they exercise uncontrollable dominion over the conduct. This is the case sometimes during the whole attack, and at others only during particular paroxysms : in either of these cases, the actions are entirely out of the control of the patients, and of course they are not morally responsible for them. They are frequently most opposite to the usual habits of the patient, and this is the natural consequence of the powerful excitement of one set of feelings, whilst those which in a healthy state counteract and regulate their action, are comparatively dormant. But in many cases, those who are really insane on some subjects, are as capable of distinguishing between right and wrong as the sane. I remember a patient, who was at work with a sharp instrument, telling me, in a fit of passion, that " if he killed me he knew he should not suffer for it, because he was mad." From my knowledge of the man's disposition, I had no fear of such a catastrophe : but if violence be committed under such circumstances, is it consistent with common sense, that the man should be considered not a responsible being, because he happens to have some erroneous notions about property, and fancies that he is entitled to an estate which belongs to another? Where the act is the result of the disease, the case is perfectly different. Martin, whose mind was morbidly impressed with the notion, that it was his duty to burn York Minster, was justly acquitted on the ground of his insanity. In many of the insane, there is a great combination of moral evil with cerebral disorder ; and it is exceedingly difficult to distinguish between that which is the result merely of vice and perverseness, and that which is the consequence of disease. Where it is clear that an improper act arises solely from wickedness, the patient ought to be dealt with as a moral agent, and its recurrence should be prevented by making it understood that repetition will be attended with some positive inconvenience, or with the deprivation of some enjoyment. But we must remember, with the insane as well as with the sane, that although fear of punishment, moral discipline, and the experience of the present advantages of virtuous conduct will do much to check the actual indulgence in vicious propensities, yet nothing but religion, and the operation of the Spirit of God upon the heart can eradicate the evil inclinations.

The two following examples will make the distinction, which I have endeavoured to draw between vicious and insane acts, perfectly intelligible. A young man, who had been respectably brought up, was engaged in the wine trade, a business which affords considerable temptation to intemperance : he unfortunately indulged in his potations to such an extent that he brought on a low degree of delirium tremens. Whilst under the influence of this disease he procured a pistol, as it subsequently appeared, without any evil design, but from mere folly ; and he went to see a young woman with whom he was acquainted : he was refused admission into the house, and, acting under the excitement caused by the diseased action of the brain, he fired at the person who came to the door. Happily he missed her, and the ball was found in the door-post. He was tried for the offence, and although, after he recovered from the attack of delirium tremens, he never exhibited the slightest symptom of insanity, he was, and very properly, if the distinction previously pointed out be correct, acquitted on the ground of insanity. The act in this instance arose purely from the morbid irritability of the brain, produced by disease. If it had been the result of intoxication, according to the distinction pointed out in the second chapter, as the immediate cause of the act would then have been in his own power, he must have been dealt with as responsible for it. The delirium tremens was the immediate cause of the act; but this was a permanent one, and not within his own control; although it is quite true that this continuous cause might have been avoided, had the young man not been guilty of excess. On his acquittal he was ordered into confinement, where, I believe, he remains to this day.

The other case is of a very different complexion. A man had a quarrel with his employer; he thought himself much injured by him, and he had no means of redress. This man also procured a pistol, which he carefully kept about him for some days: he met the gentleman, fired at him, and wounded him, though not mortally. He was immediately taken into custody, and subsequently tried. He exhibited much of the recklessness which is often seen to follow the gratification of revenge, but, if the report of the trial be to be depended upon, no symptoms whatever of any diseased action of the brain. As this man was acquitted by the jury on the plea of insanity, I should hope that some circumstances were disclosed at the trial, with which I am unacquainted, to lead them to that verdict. But if no material facts appeared, sufficient to evidence the existence of diseased action in the brain, the conduct in this instance must, according to my notions, be traced to moral evil, and not to insanity. Is it uncharitable to think, that under the circumstances, the jury might have been led to the conclusion they came to, from the consciousness that the ground of offence, even if true to the uttermost, could not have so worked upon their minds as to have led to so sanguinary a result; and that they consequently conceived, that any man, who permitted so trifling a cause to lead to so outrageous an act, must have been insane? The fallacy of such a mode of reasoning has already been pointed out.

CHAPTER X.

CONCLUSION.

FROM what has been already said on the subject, it appears that Insanity may be traced to three classes of causes,—viz. direct physical injuries of the brain, over-excitement from moral causes, and diseased action in it from sympathy with some other part of the body. It becomes a matter of very serious inquiry to ascertain how far the circumstances which produce it, are either directly or remotely under our control. The instinctive dread of pain possessed by man, in common with other animals, is a sufficient guarantee for his using the greatest care to avoid the accidents which are likely to expose him to an attack of insanity from the first set of causes. The only means by which his liability to suffer from these could be diminished, would be by giving him more information as to the effects likely to be produced on the system by particular circumstances, in order to induce a greater caution on his part not to place himself where he is likely to be exposed to their injurious operation. Thus, in the case previously referred to, if the man who ran without his hat, exposed to a burning sun, had known enough of the structure of his body to have been aware that he was incurring great risk of an attack of phrenitis or of insanity, he would have preferred the lesser inconvenience of being too late for the coach, and would have preserved his reason. Something also might be done habitually to strengthen that faculty which is usually called presence of mind. Many of the accidents which destroy life, or injure the limbs, might be avoided by coolness ; and this is, to a very great degree, to be acquired by education. What makes the difference in this respect between the sailor and the manmilliner ? The fact, that the latter is not called upon to rely upon his own exertions in cases of sudden danger; whilst the former, from being obliged from early life constantly to exercise his coolness in cases of emergency, acquires such a habit of self-possession and confidence in his own powers, that he can actually pass through perils with comparatively little risk to himself, which would overwhelm the other. But the cases of insanity arising from direct physical injuries are comparatively few, and but little can be done to avoid their occurrence : those which have their origin from moral causes are by far more numerous, and fortunately much more capable of being avoided : they are generally the result of our having an undue estimate of the things of this life.

Let us, by way of illustration, briefly trace the progress of the operation on the mind, of a sudden reverse of fortune, one of the most usual of the moral causes of insanity. We will suppose that this has overtaken a man from circumstances entirely out of his power, although if it be inquired into, it will be found, that it frequently arises from the neglect of that commandment, which bids us not to make haste to be rich. Now if the mind be well disciplined, the wealth, which is no longer possessed, has not been an object of inordinate affection; it has been habitually viewed as a talent, for the right use of which a great responsibility is incurred: and the mere loss of it creates no excessive uneasiness; and even if its absence affects the personal comfort of those who are the dearest, this is submitted to with a full reliance, that it is ordered by a wise and merciful Providence, whose dealings with all his creatures are exactly such as are the most conducive to their real welfare. Under these circumstances, there would not be such an anxiety as to prevent sleep, and produce an excessive sanguineous action in the brain, to terminate in insanity. The mind would be kept in peace. But let us suppose, that such a reverse has happened to one who has looked upon riches, and the pleasures to be procured by them, as the chief good; and whose life and powers, mental and bodily, have been constantly absorbed in their acquisition. To such an individual,—and unfortunately there are very many with whom this is the case,—the mere probability of the loss of that which he holds the dearest, produces a restlessness and anxiety, which weaken the nervous system, and incapacitate it from bearing up against the shock which he feels, when that which he most valued is suddenly torn out of his grasp. It cannot be a matter of surprise, that the mind not knowing where to look for consolation, should be overwhelmed, and that insanity should be the result. And we may, in a similar manner, trace to an over-estimate of the things of this life, insanity arising from loss of children, disappointed ambition,—in fact from any other moral cause. But this, painful as it is, is the result of the previous habits and conduct. With a view of making the nature of the evil more intelligible, it will be worth while to prosecute the inquiry a little further, and to endeavour to trace these habits to their origin. We shall find, that from infancy to manhood, the usual process of education is to foster that erroneous estimate of temporal things which is the general source of insanity from moral causes, and to weaken and predispose the body for its reception; unfortunately the same system prevails with both sexes. In infancy, in the higher ranks of life, the child is in a great measure left to the tuition of ignorant nurse-maids; and in many cases, with the first dawn of reason, it imbibes false and superstitious impressions, which are a source of torment to it for years; and when the child is more immediately under the presence and management of its parents, the first lesson that is impressed upon its mind, is that the gratification of the senses is the chief good. And this too is not taught in the dull, uninteresting, formal manner, in which at a much later period, and after this principle has been well ingrafted, valuable truths are attempted to be imparted. This is instilled by practice and example. In females, the next principle which is systematically brought into exercise, is vanity. As soon as the child can speak, and is capable of understanding any thing, it is taught to set a high value upon its dress: the attention is directed to it, and from early infancy, it engrosses a considerable portion of its time and thought. After the principles of love of animal gratification, and in females the love of approbation, have been carefully fostered, the next step is to provide some education for the intellect. The two classes of motives which are acted upon, are fear and emulation. The natural result of the former, with many, is to produce excess of timidity, dissimulation, and the other vices attendant upon an undue exercise of the organs of caution and secretiveness; and the inevitable consequences of the latter are, to foster selfishness. The reward of success is a personal gratification, exactly in proportion to the superiority over others. The result is an over-value of the praise and good opinion of others: this is one of the most prolific sources of suffering which the human mind can possibly feel; and it is also one of

the greatest preventives to a man's daring independently to do that which his conscience teaches
him to be right. Hence also results an excessive
activity in a set of feelings which, when over-
excited in after life, frequently terminate in insanity.
So far then as the training affects the sentiment, it is
from infancy prejudicial: it tends to foster the natural
desire for the gratification of appetite, to induce
inordinate ambition, and to create an over-estimate of wealth, and of the things of time and sense ;
and in all these points it directly leads to insanity.
It is also physically injurious, from causing at too
early a period, excess of vascular action in the brain.
The intellect is, by fear of disgrace, and hope of
praise, stimulated to an unhealthy activity. The
brain and nervous system absorb the blood, which
ought in youth to be directed to the supply of proper
muscular volume and energy. Females suffer in
this respect more than males ; in fact, the entire
want of proper exercise, and the excessive stimulus
given to the mental faculties so affect the frame,
that there is hardly a female, educated in the board-
ing-schools conducted on the usual principles, whose
spine is not more or less distorted. It is foreign
to the object of the present work to inquire,
whether this enormous expenditure of constitution,
for the sake of intellect, is most judiciously laid out
in securing the most valuable mental attainments.
It is perfectly obvious, that even if it be, a system
of education, which entirely neglects, as one of its

primary objects, the imbuing the mind with right motives, and with a due estimate of the real value of the things of this life, leaves it exposed to such excessive anxiety, on any reverse or disappointment, as tends to insanity. How little too is the real welfare usually considered in the selection of a walk in life! A combination of circumstances affording a probability of the acquisition of wealth, is usually the only guide; and, with both sexes, marriages are entered into or avoided on the same principle.—But the tracing the influence of education and the habits of society, in producing insanity, would form an ample subject for another volume. The evil would be prevented by a simple obedience to the precepts of the Gospel.

In many cases, insanity arising from sympathy is entirely brought on by bad management of the constitution: independently of those instances where it is the result of obvious excess, it frequently arises from a very slight moral cause, acting upon a highly irritable nervous system, habitually too much excited by the use of stimulus. Indeed, as has been previously observed, the constant use of any stimulus ought, if possible, to be avoided by those who have a predisposition to the disease. In fact any circumstances, which tend to put the body out of order, ought to be guarded against; and much of insanity might be avoided, if a practical knowledge of the human frame, and of the influence of external circumstances upon it, were made a branch of education, both amongst males and females. Indeed I am convinced, that with very few exceptions, a right and religious disciplining of the mind, with a judicious and careful selection of the walk in life, and a prudent management of the body, would exempt mankind from the horrors of this painful and mysterious disease.

APPENDIX.

APPENDIX.

NOTE.—Page 97.

MASTURBATION, the cause alluded to, is a fertile source of insanity. I have no hesitation in saying, that in a very large number of patients in all public asylums, the disease may be attributed to that cause. The general debility, which is produced by this disgusting habit, is more severely felt in the brain and nervous system in some constitutions than in others; and whilst a pale face, general lassitude, drowsiness, cold extremities, trembling hands, and a voracious appetite, are the indications of its existence in one, the brain is the first part to give way in another, and insanity takes place. We must not, however, omit to mention that the practice is often the consequence, as well as the cause of the disease. I have no doubt, that when from any circumstance the cerebellum becomes in a high state of excitement, venereal desires are the result, and this practice is too often resorted to.

NOTE.—Page 133.

When in incipient insanity, or in particular exacerbations in chronic cases, an excess of libidinous feeling is exhibited, this is almost the only premonitory symptom. The cerebellum is the part where the greatest heat is to be found. Indeed, whilst the other part of the scalp remains of its natural temperature, this is often found excessively hot, and, perceptibly to the touch, of a greater heat than the parts of the body under the clothes.

We have a case in the Asylum at the present time of a young man, about twenty-eight years of age, who has been insane several years. He is naturally very libidinous, but exacerbation of these feelings comes on periodically. He is generally occupied as a shoemaker, and is industrious. The first premonitory symptom is a degree of restlessness and unwillingness to work. This is followed by his endeavouring to expose his person, and take improper liberties with any of the female servants who may have occasion to pass through the ward.

On his head being carefully examined the other day by my colleague, Dr. Button, and myself, in going through the ward, the whole of the back part of it and the neck were found to be considerably hotter than any other part, not only of the head, but even of the chest under his clothes.

Shaving the head, cupping, and cold applications, with small doses of nitre and of tartar emetic, materially tend to abate the paroxysm ; and I have no doubt that, in a few days, he will be in his ordinary state of health.

NOTE.—Page 136.

Cases of insanity arising from masturbation are most easily distinguishable from the appearance of the countenance, to those thoroughly conversant with the disease ; yet any attempt to describe the particular symptoms would be more likely to mislead than to be of any practical utility. It is probable that, in these cases, the cerebrum is weakened from the due supply of blood being withdrawn from it, and forced into other parts of the body ; and probably, also, from the cerebellum engrossing more than its share.

NOTE.—Page 145.

By far the most frequent cause of fatuity is debility of the brain and nervous system, from the cerebrum not receiving a due proportion of blood for the carrying on its functions, in consequence of the pernicious habit of masturbation. In the natural and healthy condition of man, every thing is so well ordered, that each part receives the due share of blood requisite for its nutrition, and for the performance of its regular and appointed functions. But man has, to a considerable extent, the power of increasing the rapidity of the circulation, either generally throughout the system, as by fermented liquors, or partially through particular portions of it, as by the excessive exertion of the part.

Where the circulation is only accelerated through certain portions of the body, the mass of blood not being increased, the other parts are robbed of their due share, and their functions are consequently weakened and disturbed. But as over-exercise does not generally afford gratification, this excessive voluntary circulation through particular parts of the body rarely takes place, except in the brain, where it produces insanity and the results already described, and in the parts which are affected by venery and masturbation.

It is the latter practice which is most to be dreaded and deprecated ; and however revolting to the feelings it may be to enter upon such a subject, it cannot be passed over in silence without a great violation of duty. Unhappily, it has not hitherto been exhibited in the awful light in which it deserves to be shown. A great deal has been said on dementia by previous writers on insanity ; but this, the true cause of its origin in by far the greater number of cases, has not been mentioned. It is often begun in very early youth : I have had under my care a child almost in a state of fatuity from this cause, at ten years of age, but who subsequently recovered ; and I have recently been informed, on authority, the accuracy of which I cannot doubt, of similar effects being produced from the same cause in a child not more than eight years old. In the present artificial state of society, where marriages are too frequently prevented only from the want of what are considered sufficient pecuniary means, and where scenes of dissipation are prevalent, and a highly stimulating and exciting mode of living is adopted, this vice, as it might be expected, is unfortunately continued in after life.

Independent of this dreadful disease, of which it is alone frequently the cause, there are many others which may fairly be attributed to this practice ; they do not, however, fall within the province of this work. If the dread of falling a martyr to this worst form in which it ends should deter from the practice, all the rest will be escaped.

The worst of it is, it is seldom suspected. There are many pale faces and languid and nervous feelings attributed to other causes, when all the mischief lies here ; and, when it is suspected, it is so delicate and painful a subject that it can scarcely be hinted at without a blush. It should not, however, be forgotten, that a great deal of misery in life, and insanity and premature death, is often the consequence ; and it therefore demands some sacrifice of feeling, especially from those who have the charge of youth : they ought to be warned, indirectly at least, of the consequences. It is seldom, in these cases, that any one faculty is observed to be more weakened than the rest ; there is no particular chord that on being touched denotes disorder, but a general languor and inability for either mental or bodily exertion. The exhaustion often occasions a great desire for food, and a large quantity is often taken, though there is no corresponding healthy appearance from it ; it is also attended with much drowsiness and irritability if roused, till death puts an end to the scene. Whenever I hear of these symptoms coming on, without any known hereditary or moral cause, I begin to suspect that something is wrong here. It is practised, too, by those who little think of its fatal results ; by persons otherwise most exemplary, and considered so highly moral, that any cause is looked for, as the occasion of the symptoms observed, rather than the real one. I have frequently been fortunate enough to detect it in time ; and, upon mentioning my suspicions, have had them confirmed by the parties, who themselves little suspected the cause. Some time ago I was consulted, by letter, on a case of this kind, of a young gentleman residing in Cambridge ; I communicated my suspicion to his friend, who at once told him my opinion : he acknowledged the truth of it, left off the practice, and in a month afterwards I had the satisfaction of hearing he was quite well. I wish I could add, that young *gentlemen* were the only transgressors. I hope I have said enough on this delicate and painful subject to excite that attention and alarm which its importance demands.

The lassitude and general weakness of the brain from this cause gradually increase, the patient becomes fatuous, and dies.

NOTE.—Page 244.

It has been already stated, that the cases here referred to are much more numerous than it is generally supposed. Before the patients are taken to a Lunatic Asylum the disease has usually proceeded to a direful extent ; the first stage has passed away, and it has become one of such pure debility that invigorating means only are left to us. But it is lamentable to state how little hope there is of stopping its progress : the functions of the mind have usually become so torpid that all moral reasoning has lost its effect ; and, unless the practice is discontinued, no medical means can produce the least alleviation of the symptoms, and I have been unable to discover any mode of confinement which will effectually prevent it. When in Paris, I accidentally met a French surgeon, Monsieur A. Gerentet, who then resided in the Palais Royal, No. 36 : he informed me that he had discovered an effectual mechanical preventive, and he promised to come to Hanwell and bring some of his fasteners with him. He has not yet fulfilled his promise. I have recently been informed that he has been in London, and that his contrivance is valuable : when I saw him he had not one made, and I understand from him, that, in order to be of any use, they must be fitted for the particular person intended to wear them. If the patient is alive to the deplorable consequences already caused by the practice, and to those still worse, which are to follow from its continuance, so as to be induced to abstain from it, he may generally be restored. To assist his good resolution he ought, on going to bed every night, to have his hands secured. He should sleep upon a hard mattress, without curtains, and the room should be particularly airy. Cold ablutions about the genitals and loins should be constantly applied, and he should take exercise in the open air; the diet should be nutritious, and the bowels should be kept moderately open by cooling aperients: but the Tincture of Cantharides is the most efficacious means of cure. I have long been in the habit of giving this medicine in doses of from twenty to thirty drops three times a day, increasing or diminishing them according to their effect. These patients usually exhibit great symptoms of debility, depressed spirits, a pale, languid countenance, a weak, quick pulse, cold clammy perspiration on the skin, and particularly on the hands; great drowsiness, and often a voracious appetite. After the cantharides have been continued some time, provided the previous habit is actually left off, the cerebrum and other parts of the body are again supplied with their due share of blood, the general health and spirits begin to rally; and, with them, the functions of the mind resume their accustomed power.

Diet Table.

BREAD.—14 oz. daily for each patient.

BREAKFAST.

$1\frac{1}{2}$ pint of rice, or oatmeal gruel, as is deemed most conducive to health. This is made in the following manner:—2 gallons of milk, 2 gallons of water, $2\frac{3}{4}$ pounds of oatmeal or rice, and a $\frac{1}{4}$ pound of wheat-flower, are boiled together one hour.

DINNER.

Sunday.—Roast beef; 6 oz. uncooked meat, free from bone; 4 oz. yeast dumpling, with the addition of 6 oz. vegetables. Sometimes potatoes are substituted for the dumplings.

Tuesday.—Same as on Sunday, except that boiled mutton is substituted for the beef.

Thursday.—Boiled pork instead of beef.

Saturday.—14 oz. pie, made of the coarse beef, with potatoes.

Soup, made from the meat boiled the day before, with the bones stewed, thickened with barley, rice, peas, and vegetables, and flavoured with onions, pot-herbs, and cayenne pepper, forms their dinners on the other days of the week.

SUPPER.
Same as breakfast.

As the season affords, the patients are sometimes indulged with fruit pies : and every Christmas they participate in the usual festivity of roast beef and plum-pudding.

BEER.—One half-pint is the daily allowance at dinner for the industrious and infirm. The healthy, who do not work, are not allowed malt liquor. Those who labour out of doors, or are really efficient in the wards, also receive one-third of a pint of beer at eleven in the morning, and the same quantity at four in the afternoon.

Many of the patients, who are engaged in the domestic offices, receive indulgences ; and several, who assist the servants, sit up and partake with them of supper. Various extras for the sick are also allowed : but their rations are not stopped, and, as they are frequently unable to participate in them, it necessarily increases the allowance for the actual consumers. In fact, this is sufficient, but I do not think, superfluous.

RULES AND REGULATIONS

To be Printed, and hung up in each Keeper's and Servant's Room.

First.—Every patient on admission is to be stripped and washed, and it is to be carefully observed if there be any swelling in any part of the body, vermin, or spots on the skin; the hair is to be cut close and combed, and the patient is then to be clothed in the asylum dress.

Second.—Every keeper and servant is expected to rise at six o'clock; the keepers will then immediately wash and comb their patients, and observe if there be any soreness or discoloration of the skin in any part of the body. They are expected also to examine the stools and urine of the patients, so as to be able to report their state, and every other particular concerning them. On any patient appearing ill, information is immediately to be taken of it to the apothecary's shop. They must also pay the strictest attention to the administering of the medicines, &c. agreeably to the directions.

Third.—When the bell rings for prayers, they will attend with such patients as are in a proper state. At eight o'clock the patients will breakfast; as soon as breakfast is over, the keepers will clean out the galleries and bed-rooms, lay the beds and bedding to air, and remove the wet straw and every kind of dirt or dirty linen, and, in fine weather, open the windows. It must be understood, that no place will be considered *clean* which can be made *cleaner*.

Fourth.—The patients will dine at one o'clock, and sup at seven. They will go to bed as soon as supper is over, and no clothing is to be allowed to remain in the room. One hour before every meal, the keepers will take down their trays and tins to the kitchens, and at the same time take from the apothecary's shop the medicines ordered for their patients; and when the bell rings (but not before) the keepers, with a patient to assist them, will go to their respective kitchens for the provisions. After each meal, the dishes, trenchers, kits, &c. are to be carefully washed, and every knife, fork, and spoon is to be counted, and locked up. The male keepers will shave their patients on Wednesdays and Saturdays.

Fifth.—The keepers will not be permitted to leave their ward except at the time appointed above, unless some very urgent business demand it, when he or she will inform the keeper in the next ward of the cause of their absence; but they must, at no time whatever, leave their wards without having first locked up in their rooms, any patients who are liable to be violent, or strike another, excepting such patient is properly secured. Any male keeper wanting any thing from the housekeeper or kitchen, must apply in the office. No patient to be allowed either to deliver out the meat, beer, bread, or pottage, to the patients. No patient to be permitted to leave the wards in the morning, before breakfast, to assist the house-servants, without the servants personally fetching them. No patient to be allowed to fetch either medicine, wine, or beer, from the apothecary's shop.

Sixth.—The keepers are to be accountable for all bed and other linen, the patients' clothing, and the various articles belonging to the wards.

Seventh.—Any keeper striking or ill-treating a patient will, for the first offence, be fined five shillings, and be dismissed for the second; nor are the keepers to use any harsh or intemperate language, which tends to irritate or disturb them, as their duty is uniformly to be discharged in a mild, humane manner. They are at all times to appear clean and tidy in their persons, and strictly decorous in their behaviour.

Eighth.—Any keeper found making a perquisite of any kind, or selling any thing to a patient, will be fined five shillings for the first offence, and dismissed for the second. Any servant, from whose custody a patient escapes, through negligence, shall pay such proportion of the expense of retaking the patient, as the magistrates at their next meeting shall order.

Ninth.—On Saturday, at eight o'clock in the morning, every keeper is expected to deliver a list, in writing, of the household utensils wanted in his or her ward for the following week, which will be delivered on the Monday morning. If at any time a knife, instrument, or tool, such as a brush, fire-irons, &c. shall be left unlocked up after using, or the door of the fire-guards left unlocked, each keeper shall forfeit a shilling. Any keeper leaving his or her ward or airing court, without giving notice to the keeper in the next ward, where he or she is gone, shall forfeit one shilling; and any keeper permitting a patient to get up, and go about the ward or house, before he or she is up to take charge of, or deliver the patient to the care of others, shall forfeit one shilling.

Tenth.—No person or relative, calling to see any keeper or servant, will be allowed to go into the kitchen or wards, but must remain in the receiving room appropriated for the males, on the east, and females on the west sides of the house. Each and every keeper, and out-door servant, to attend at prayers every evening, in the chapel, at half-past nine o'clock precisely, or forfeit sixpence each, for each default. It is expected that every keeper or nurse will examine the water taps in their wards, immediately after putting the patients to bed, so that no water be wasted, or forfeit five shillings.

THE END.

R. CLAY, PRINTER, BREAD-STREET-HILL.

Classics in Psychiatry

An Arno Press Collection

American Psychiatrists Abroad. 1975

Arnold, Thomas. **Observations On The Nature, Kinds, Causes, And Prevention Of Insanity.** 1806. Two volumes in one

Austin, Thomas J. **A Practical Account Of General Paralysis, Its Mental And Physical Symptoms, Statistics, Causes, Seat, And Treatment.** 1859

Bayle, A[ntoine] L[aurent] J[esse]. **Traité Des Maladies Du Cerveau Et De Ses Membranes.** 1826

Binz, Carl. **Doctor Johann Weyer.** 1896

Blandford, G. Fielding. **Insanity And Its Treatment.** 1871

Bleuler, Eugen. **Textbook Of Psychiatry.** 1924

Braid, James. **Neurypnology.** 1843

Brierre de Boismont, A[lexandre-Jacques-François]. **Hallucinations.** 1853

Brown, Mabel Webster, compiler. **Neuropsychiatry And The War:** A Bibliography With Abstracts and **Supplement I,** October 1918. Two volumes in one

Browne, W. A. F. **What Asylums Were, Are, And Ought To Be.** 1837

Burrows, George Man. **Commentaries On The Causes, Forms, Symptoms And Treatment, Moral And Medical, Of Insanity.** 1828

Calmeil, L[ouis]-F[lorentin]. **De La Folie:** Considérée Sous Le Point De Vue Pathologique, Philosophique, Historique Et Judiciaire, Depuis La Renaissance Des Sciences En Europe Jusqu'au Dix-Neuvième Siècle. 1845. Two volumes in one

Calmeil, L[ouis] F[lorentin]. **De La Paralysie Considérée Chez Les Aliénés.** 1826

Dejerine, J[oseph Jules] and E. Gauckler. **The Psychoneuroses And Their Treatment By Psychotherapy.** [1913]

Dunbar, [Helen] Flanders. **Emotions And Bodily Changes.** 1954

Ellis, W[illiam] C[harles]. **A Treatise On The Nature, Symptoms, Causes And Treatment Of Insanity.** 1838

Emminghaus, H[ermann]. **Die Psychischen Störungen Des Kindesalters.** 1887

Esdaile, James. **Mesmerism In India,** And Its Practical Application In Surgery And Medicine. 1846

Esquirol, E[tienne]. **Des Maladies Mentales.** 1838. Three volumes in two

Feuchtersleben, Ernst [Freiherr] von. **The Principles Of Medical Psychology.** 1847

Georget, [Etienne-Jean]. **De La Folie:** Considérations Sur Cette Maladie. 1820

Haslam, John. **Observations On Madness And Melancholy.** 1809

Hill, Robert Gardiner. **Total Abolition Of Personal Restraint In The Treatment Of The Insane.** 1839

Janet, Pierre [Marie-Felix] and F. Raymond. **Les Obsessions Et La Psychasthénie.** 1903. Two volumes

Janet, Pierre [Marie-Felix]. **Psychological Healing.** 1925. Two volumes

Kempf, Edward J. **Psychopathology.** 1920

Kraepelin, Emil. **Manic-Depressive Insanity And Paranoia.** 1921

Kraepelin, Emil. **Psychiatrie:** Ein Lehrbuch Für Studirende Und Aerzte. 1896

Laycock, Thomas. **Mind And Brain.** 1860. Two volumes in one

Liébeault, A[mbroise]-A[uguste]. **Le Sommeil Provoqué Et Les États Analogues.** 1889

Mandeville, B[ernard] De. **A Treatise Of The Hypochondriack And Hysterick Passions.** 1711

Morel, B[enedict] A[ugustin]. **Traité Des Degénérescences Physiques, Intellectuelles Et Morales De L'Espèce Humaine.** 1857. Two volumes in one

Morison, Alexander. **The Physiognomy Of Mental Diseases.** 1843

Myerson, Abraham. **The Inheritance Of Mental Diseases.** 1925

Perfect, William. **Annals Of Insanity.** [1808]

Pinel, Ph[ilippe]. **Traité Médico-Philosophique Sur L'Aliénation Mentale.** 1809

Prince, Morton, et al. **Psychotherapeutics.** 1910

Psychiatry In Russia And Spain. 1975

Ray, I[saac]. **A Treatise On The Medical Jurisprudence Of Insanity.** 1871

Semelaigne, René. **Philippe Pinel Et Son Oeuvre Au Point De Vue De La Médecine Mentale.** 1888

Thurnam, John. **Observations And Essays On The Statistics Of Insanity.** 1845

Trotter, Thomas. **A View Of The Nervous Temperament.** 1807

Tuke, D[aniel] Hack, editor. **A Dictionary Of Psychological Medicine.** 1892. Two volumes

Wier, Jean. **Histoires, Disputes Et Discours Des Illusions Et Impostures Des Diables, Des Magiciens Infames, Sorcieres Et Empoisonneurs.** 1885. Two volumes

Winslow, Forbes. **On Obscure Diseases Of The Brain And Disorders Of The Mind.** 1860

Burdett, Henry C. **Hospitals And Asylums Of The World.** 1891-93. Five volumes. 2,740 pages on NMA standard 24x-98 page microfiche only